# So You Want to Lose Weight and Keep It Off?

## Do It Your Way!

**By: Jeff Gold**

So You Want to Lose Weight After 50? Do It Your Way!

"It is not the critic who counts; not the man who points out how the strong man stumbles, or where the doer of deeds could have done them better. The credit belongs to the man who is actually in the arena, whose face is marred by dust and sweat and blood; who strives valiantly; who errs, who comes short again and again, because there is no effort without error and shortcoming; but who does actually strive to do the deeds; who knows great enthusiasms, the great devotions; who spends himself in a worthy cause; who at the best knows in the end the triumph of high achievement, and who at the worst, if he fails, at least fails while daring greatly, so that his place shall never be with those cold and timid souls who neither know victory nor defeat."

Theodore Roosevelt, 1910

Disclaimer

The following viewpoints in this book are those of Jeff Gold. These views are based on his personal experiences over his lifetime.

The intention of this book is to entertain and share his story about losing weight and the challenges he had his entire life losing weight.

This is not a medical guide, nor is it medical research. All attempts have been made to verify the information provided by this publication. Neither the author, the publisher, or anyone named in this publication assumes any responsibility for errors, omissions, or contrary interpretations of the subject matter herein.

The author does not recommend or endorse any product, video, or person. Any references to products or persons are simply to let the reader know what products the author uses or persons that the author has been exposed to. The reader is strongly encouraged to do his or her own research and to consult a medical professional in every step of the weight loss process.

This book is for entertainment purposes only. The views expressed are those of the author alone and should not be taken as expert instruction or commands. The reader is responsible for his or her future action. This book makes no guarantees of weight loss or of health benefits. You should always consult a medical provider who is a medical doctor before taking any supplement or changing your health habits. Working with your medical provider is a must.

Neither the author nor the publisher assumes any responsibility or liability on the behalf of the purchaser or reader of these materials.

The views expressed are based on his personal experiences in a lifetime of weight loss.

To those who I could never thank enough: To all those who noticed I lost weight and congratulated me. Noticing that someone has lost weight and telling them is the motivation to continue. Thank you! My wife Shawn, who through her terrible battle with cancer, I finally found the strength to battle my disease and addiction of overeating and living an unhealthy lifestyle of eating fast food and junk food. Through all Shawn has gone through, her priority was taking care of her family and mostly me. I have never seen anyone go through the years of pain and treatment without complaining or even once outwardly feeling sorry for herself. She is my inspiration to be as driven as I am. I love you more than anything!

Table of Contents

*Podcast Invitation*

I want to invite you to listen to the So You Want to Lose Weight podcast. We speak with others in the same battle to lose weight and live a happier and healthier lifestyle.

*Social Media*

Please visit our Facebook page at So You Want to Lose Weight? Jeff gives updates about the book and other information in the weight loss journey.

# Introduction

It's always been said that losing weight after 50 is harder and yes, it is. I lost 50 pounds in the eight months prior to my 55th birthday, which seems great, but I used to lose 50 pounds in as little as three months when I was younger. In fact, I once went from over 240 pounds to 167 pounds in six months to win a weight loss contest and to complete in a martial arts tournament at a lighter weight classification. I have never had a problem losing weight and I have definitely never had a problem gaining it back. So, as the clock ticked past the 50 year point in my life, I never worried about that extra 10-15 pounds a year I was putting on. I would simply cut back on the food and work out like crazy just like I did every other time in my life, but this time it was different, now I am over 50!

I have heard the saying, "50 is the new 40" and there is even a movie "50 is the new 30," but I haven't watched it. I do not know about all this, but I can tell you this much, I am 55 and I am not what I was at 40 and definitely not what I was at 30! Now don't get me wrong, I am in decent health compared to a lot of people in my age group and I am definitely more active and working than most my age, but I do feel the years, especially in my joints. I originally titled this book, "So You Want to Lose Weight Over 50?" I found the majority of people asking me how I lost the weight and then asking how I keep it off while still eating what I do were well under 50 years old. For me, the challenges were being over 50 and losing weight, but the challenge for everyone is keeping it off after you lose it. This is the real fight and hopefully I have found a way to stay in it for all the rounds, not just the first few.

This book is a journey through one of the most difficult times in my life and a lot of changes that had to be made, not just for me, but for my family. There are countless numbers of books on weight loss and many great doctors and health professionals that tell you exactly what to do to lose weight and be a healthier you. I know, I have read many books and tried many different diets over my half century on this fragile earth. I am not a medical doctor, though I am finishing my doctorate in education and healthcare administration as I am writing this book. I do have a fairly good background in the general field of healthcare with over 30 years in emergency medicine as a firefighter and paramedic. I have an undergraduate degree in emergency medical services, I went to nursing school with my wife, and most importantly, good old life experience. The information contained in this book is for entertainment purposes and you should always consult with a medical doctor before starting any diet, exercise program, or supplement program. Throughout my life I have worked in a multitude of high risk jobs that required me to have yearly physicals, blood draws, and cardiac stress tests. Most people do not have these type of medical tests performed unless there is a problem. We always hear about people who are young and drop of a massive heart attack while they are playing sports or mowing their lawn. I wonder if they had these advanced tests on an annual basis would they still be here? So check with your doctor and make sure you are able to take on a new exercise regimen or diet program. I consulted with my personal physician just about every step of my weight loss journey and most importantly, I listened to his advice and did what he recommended. I also realized that doctors are human and they do not know everything and most do not go home at night and study new medical findings until they fall asleep and start the next day seeing patients again. The field of medicine is constantly changing and evolving and this is why it is important to have a good doctor. This and many other areas you may never have thought of will be discussed in my journey to losing weight and keeping it off, so enjoy!

# Chapter 1

## Starting Out

Most diets I have seen start hard at first. You count down to the start of a diet like it's the end of freedom and in a way, it is. You cannot eat what you want, you probably have to change your schedule around to exercise, and you are probably going to be hungry and miserable. So why do we do this to ourselves? Maybe this is the reason why almost half of all dieters quit in the first week. Think about it, if you are used to taking in 4,000 calories or more and then you try to cut down to 1,500 calories immediately, you are going to be miserable. So start off slowly reducing your calories the first week and start making those changes in your diet at your own pace.

You always hear that breakfast is the most important meal of the day and I never followed that advice until I decided to lose and keep it off. Being the busy person I am I always relied on a high carb and caffeine filled breakfast to get me started. I would usually grab some prepackaged breakfast snack on the way out with my Diet Mt. Dew and then head to my local mega gas station and get my favorite meal of two pieces of meat lover's pizza. I would get the largest fountain drink and mix regular Mt. Dew and Diet Mt. Dew to get that extra sugar boost and eat it on the way to work. I can only guess I was taking in over 150 carbs and probably 10 times that in calories, but it woke me up and I felt full and happy. Sometimes for lunch I would get a Zaxby's salad because it seemed healthy, but it was almost 700 calories and I always added extra ranch dressing and had a Coke because they did not serve Mt. Dew. Diner was usually eating out or something with rice or pasta. So, I was in keeping with the typical American calorie intake of around 3,600 calories a day, or well past that.

Of all the foods available in this great county, my favorite to eat at home or to order out is the good old American hamburger. Unlike my dad who ate a McDonald's hamburger every day of his life, I wanted a thick burger with a thick-soft toasted bun and extra ketchup to dip it in. I would eat a McDonald's burger, but it was a double cheeseburger and I usually had two. I would take in 900 calories for the two doubles, then fries, and of course a large Coke, since they don't serve Diet Mt. Dew. I had to find a way of making this into something I could enjoy, yet still lose weight.

Over the years, the diet that has always worked for me was a higher intake of protein than carbohydrates. This was prior to the "Keto and Carnivore Diets" becoming popular. I just experimented and found that it worked. I knew that if I cut the carbs out completely I would have side effects like headaches, loss of energy, and most likely lightheadedness. Since I had started feeling lightheaded and nauseous when I did not eat enough carbs and I was waking up in the middle of the night to eat, I knew there was a problem. This was probably pre-diabetes in the making and what I was feeling was my blood sugar dropping because I was so used to having high levels when I was eating an uncontrolled diet. When I decided to finally lose weight the right way I knew it would take a long time and that I could not get discouraged with only losing a pound or so a week.

How did I start? I decided to take my favorite meal and make it for breakfast. As is the theme of this entire book, not everything works for every person trying to lose weight and not everybody likes the same food. For me, a hamburger in the morning sounds great! For some of you, this is going to be a mortal sin not having bacon and eggs or cereal and milk. For me, this was easy. My mom never made meals, especially breakfast. I have never been a big bacon fan, which along with not drinking coffee, some people just don't understand.

I started off with a hamburger in the morning that was beneficial to have while taking vitamins and supplements. It is very important that if a vitamin or supplement says "take with food," do so. Mostly because some of these can make you nauseous and not feeling well is the opposite of what you want. My favorite bun was a soft Hawaiian style bun that I would toast with butter. I usually had fries with this, but I cut out the fries and just had a larger burger. I substituted the high carb-calorie bun with a light bun and removed a pinch of the breading at first. I recycle everything possible. I put the left over things like that into my compost pile, so in my mind, there is no waste. I used the regular mayonnaise, shredded lettuce, ketchup and substituted the fries with some potato chips. Not a whole bag of chips, about five or ten. If I could not come home for lunch, I ate something higher in protein then carbs. Sometimes I would even get my McDonald's or Burger King double cheeseburger and take the thicker bun off.

The one thing you must remember is that in this start-off week you're not going to see that big drop of weight. The first week is the hardest physically and psychologically and you want to see a big win for all that hard work. My first week of "cutting back" I only saw a two pound loss. It was a bit disappointing because I also added more physical activity. Physical activity is a huge part of losing weight. It helps you burn calories and builds muscle. Keep in mind, the muscle I am talking about is not the pumped up vein-showing muscle that we all want to have, well most guys that is. I am talking about muscle that helps us move and function. The MyFitnessPal app has a step tracker and other ways you can enter exercise and calories burned, but it is not always easy to look back at past workouts, well not for me. I use it to log in food and it shows your physical activity and compares it to the calories you take in. It's probably me, but I like easy. I walk a lot anyway, so I increased my steps daily, even if it was only a few. I try to walk every day and set a specific route and try to increase the time. I try to add more steps even if it is just walking in an area to get the steps in. I travel overseas frequently and have been stuck on 15 hour flights. I make it a point to get up and walk around the cabin, mostly when others are sleeping. Sometimes it was difficult when you are plus sized adult at near 270 pounds, but the international flights seemed to have bigger aisles. Add steps everywhere you can; park your car farther away and walk, walk a little extra in the store, and stand when you can. I try to stand as much as possible, even when I am on my computer. It is good for your back and good for your metabolism.

I go into depth about gym memberships and other workouts in Chapter 3. Many people get a gym membership when they start a diet. They hit the gym hard or start off on some advanced cardio class that makes them so sore or intimidated that they don't go back. There are a lot of online workout programs that are very good. Before these programs got popular on the internet, I lost a lot of weight doing P90X. In fact, this is when I went from around 240 pounds to 167. I felt great and for the first time in my life I could do dozens of pull-ups and what seemed to be a never ending amount of push-ups. I was also in my early 40's and I never realized what aging 15 years does to a person! Due to the injuries and ailments that caught up with me in the last 15 years, I am not able to do all the push-up and pull-ups in the workout, but still do some of the martial arts workouts. Beachbodyondemand.com has a good and large variety of online workouts with originals including P90X, Insanity, plus dozens of others. I think I pay $99 a year for it and like I have said, I do not get a cut or a sponsorship for putting the names in this book. The programs and items I mention here are what I have found in my weight loss journey. Find what works for you and start off slow. You will see the improvements at the end!

Each week I add more exercise, whether it was more steps a day or even a weekend project that keeps me moving. I worked all my life to get a swimming pool and finally decided to build the pool and patio of my dreams complete with an outside kitchen and bar. The pool was to keep me active and a swimming pool is what got me back to work after getting hit by a car in 1994. When your joints and bones hurt, the less gravity that a salt water pool gives you is great. To offset all the extra work I had to do to pay for the pool and kitchen, I did the landscaping myself. I had about 720 square foot of landscape rocks to put down, so this became my multi-weekend workout.

Without going into too much detail, because it may be one of the next series of books; So You Want to Landscape on a Budget, I did all the work myself. Instead of renting or borrowing a dump trailer or having it delivered, I picked up the rocks, 3,000 pounds at a time. Then I would drive the rocks home and unloaded the trailer full of rocks. I repeated this each weekend I didn't have to work for several months until the project was done. There is nothing like shoveling rocks in the Florida heat and humidity to give you a workout. These weekends were "hump" breakers in the sense that when I was stuck at a weight for over a week, that weekend I would burn off a ton of calories and get over the hump. I got the idea from a firefighter friend of mine who would pull weeds in his yard every day for a set amount of hours. It was a methodic exercise of bending over and squatting to pull the weeds. I finally asked him why he did not purchase a weed-killer type of fertilizer and he explained it was his workout. He listed to music and would bend at the waist for one weed and squat for the next, all the while holding his stomach muscles tight to add to the core strengthening. He lost 30 plus pounds doing this along with change in eating habits. Find something productive to do either around your house or to help others. Make it a practical exercise event. Painting a house or any type of building is an awesome exercise, especially if you are climbing a ladder to do so. If you don't believe me, watch the first Karate Kid movie or the new Cobra Kai! All joking aside, boredom leads to overeating, find something to do that is both a calorie burner and productive.

If you drink regular soda everyone will tell you to stop all together. I will never do that because I could not stop drinking Diet Mt. Dew. Even though Mt. Dew is banned in Asia and Europe because it contains Brominated Vegetable Oil or BVO that has bromine in it, I still couldn't stop drinking it. I finally did cut my beloved Diet Mt. Dew out, but I still have cravings for it. I have exchanged it for green tea, but it is not the same. I have also found that the green tea I have been drinking causes me to have a sore throat sometimes. I cannot find this happening to anyone else in my research, so I know I will need to go to the doctor. I just want more information than to be told to quit drinking it.

If you can stop drinking the sugary sodas all together, do so! If not, try diet versions, just start off on ice. Try substituting unsweetened tea or something like that. If you are from the south, "Sweet Tea" is full of sugar. I think it is all sugar with a little bit of tea in it. Tea alone or with a no-calorie sweetener is fine if you need that caffeine fix, but the traditional "Sweet Tea" with 220 calories, almost 50 carbs, and over 50 grams of sugar will not help. I drink an alkali water that one of my wife's oncologists told us it was good for boosting human immunity. I have also read the same thing about alkali water in several other sources. Wal-Mart sells their brand of alkali water and it is good for mixing various flavor packs that you can also get in the Great Value brand. I personally mix a probiotic-cherry tart and another strawberry pack together so it tastes like cherry Kool-Aid. Just be careful of the sweeteners, some have been linked to cancer. In fact, when you start researching artificial sweeteners they all seem bad, but you can't cut everything out at once.

Vitamins are important and when your body is lacking in a certain vitamin, it makes you want to take in food to feed the craving. I have tried several multi-vitamins, including the gummy ones that tasted good, but have decided to stick with Nature's Way Alive Max3 multi-vitamin. The benefit with them is that the percentages seem perfect for me, but they are larger tablets and you need to take three a day. I don't have a problem taking the larger tablets, just spreading the routine out over the day takes a while to adapt to. When starting off, don't want to buy the big bottles of supplements like I did. You will have bottles of supplements you don't in your cabinets taking up space. You hate to throw them because they cost so much, but unless a close friend wants to try them, most people feel funny about taking open bottles of pills. The big bottles seem like such a good value compared to the small ones, but it you don't take them you lost money. As you learn how your body loses weight and stays healthy you will find what works and what doesn't. I will talk more about vitamins and supplements later in Chapter 8 and it is extremely important that you have a good daily regimen of vitamins and supplements.

I listen to a lot of audio books and hopefully you do too, since I am producing several myself. I was recently listening to a book about motivation and general self-help. A suggestion that the writer gave was not to tell people you are starting a major project or life change. The reason you don't want to broadcast what you are doing is that both you and others will expect to see results. So if you don't succeed as quickly as you expect, only you will know. For me, no one really noticed my weight loss until I was down 50 pounds. Most people did not really notice my weight loss until I lost 70 pounds. I kept it to myself and denied dieting when asked. I even kept my same clothes and just took them to a tailor when they were so big that I couldn't wear them anymore. I went from a 46 inch waste to a 36 inch waist, but it took well over 18 months.

Get one scale and weigh yourself daily and record your weight. They even make a Bluetooth scale that automatically sends your weight to your smartphone, but I guess my phone is not smart enough, it doesn't work. Be ready for fluctuations in your daily weight and weigh yourself at the same time every day. I weigh myself in the morning after I wake up. I use MyFitnessPal app to log in my daily weigh and all my food. Even if I veered off course that day, I logged it in. The app will keep track of your exercise and try to bring it together to show you how to burn calories to exceed what you took in. I think a lot of it was psychological, but being honest and recording what you eat is a great way to reflect on your lifestyle.

Finally, as you may have noticed, I started out talking about calories and slowly transitioned into carbohydrates. I only count carbohydrates now. I don't care if I take in three times the recommended calorie intake for men, which is around 2,000 a day, I just watch my carb intake. What I watch is to make sure my carbs are low and my protein is high. This will be discussed in detail throughout the book.

## Chapter 2

## **Some Things You Need to Know**

I did not want to start this book off with a list of definitions and make you think it is a textbook. I am going to list out "some things" you need to know to understand the book. I will do this list of definitions in a semi-formal way that will help you understand the book. There are a lot of different diets out there and every time I try to explain what I am doing someone will reply back that I am doing "Keto" or the Carnivore Diet. So, I think it's important we know a little bit out these diets and other terms before we get into the "meat" of the book. The definitions are more of an overview from various sources instead of an official medical or dictionary definition. Everything in this book is in my own words and I strongly encourage you to research everything on your own. There are a variety of resources you can find online that are available for free. Just make sure you look at many and look for sources from true medical sources and not just someone who was previously posting "cat videos." Just because someone claims to be a doctor, look them up and find out their background and if they are a licensed medical doctor or not. Public records are a wonderful thing and each state will have information online to verify medical licensing and may even list any complaints in detail. Do you due diligence to make sure the person you are listening to is who they say they are.

Here are some phrases or diets you may hear about in this book or in your research. Remember, these descriptions are in my own words from researching various sources and you may or may not agree with my description. Please research each on your own and the products or people that may be listed are sources for you to research yourself and not the only authority on the subject.

*Adkins Diet*

The Adkins Diet was started by Dr. Robert Adkins and marketed in 1989. The accompanying book from the diet was a top seller in "fad diets." This was one of the original low-carb and high protein diets to be marketed in America. The diet was in the height of its popularity in 2003 when Dr. Adkins died of cardiac issues related to a virus. Rumors went around that it was due to his diet and combined with a law suit citing the diet caused a person to have a high LDL or bad cholesterol level, the company filed for bankruptcy. The diet is still around and operating under a different company, but the Adkins Diet and associated foods are still being sold today.

*Carnivore Diet*

The carnivore is a meat based diet without the intake of plants. One of the best explanations of the Carnivore Diet is a YouTube video by Dr. Paul Saladino titled "Debunking the Carnivore Diet." Dr. Saladino is a medical doctor and speaks about how plants can cause many issues in the human body. He also talks about a theory that plants create defense mechanisms to survive and some of these defense mechanisms can be toxic. According to his website carnivoremd.com, Dr. Saladino went to medical school at the University of Arizona and completed his residency at the University of Washington. Prior to medical school he was a physician assistant and now maintains a private practice in San Diego, California. The video mentioned above has a lot of information and the theory is interesting. There are plenty of other videos on YouTube and sites on the internet about the Carnivore Diet. Some are very strict and some are not, but most Carnivore Diets do not accept any plant based foods or supplements.

## Intermittent Fasting

This is a really vague term that can be used in several different ways. Basically, this is fasting or not eating for a significant period of the day or for multiple days. There are a few people who do really well on this, but I would not be one of them. There is a lot of research on this and if you want to look into it, please research it fully and consult your medical provider prior to starting.

## The Keto Diet

The ketogenic diet or "Keto Diet" is a high-fat, high-protein, low or no carbohydrate diet. The diet forces the body to burn fat in lieu of carbohydrates. Normally carbohydrates in food are converted into glucose, which is then transported around the body to provide energy. If there aren't a lot of carbohydrates taken in or basically none at all, the liver converts fat into fatty acids and ketone bodies. The fatty acids and ketones are used for energy to areas of the body including the brain.

The Keto Diet is well documented and a simple internet search will result in a lot of commercial programs with some pretty well known stars and atheletes that say they use it. Some say you take in one gram of protein per pound of body weight per day and limit the grams of carbohydrates o between 10 and 15 grams a day. I know people who claim they take in zero grams of carbohydrates per day. I have tried this and when I got the effects of the "Keto Flu," I stopped. The "Keto Flu" is a term that usually comes in the first few days your body goes into ketosis and basically you feel like you are getting the flu. Not a good thing during a pandemic, so I am avoiding it. Those who I know who swear by this say it goes away, but I couldn't make a full day. I still know when I haven't taken in enough carbs in a day and get that feeling. I eat some peanut butter or take a bite of my MET-RX bar and all is good within minutes. Like everything here, research this one completely and consult your medical provider before trying it.

## Low Carbohydrate Diet

The "Low Carb Diet" is a diet that revolves around carbohydrates and not calories or fats. What this means is you do not do the traditional diet of tracking calories or the calorie-in and calorie-out diet. When you eat a lot of carbohydrates your body releases insulin. When people eat a food containing carbohydrates, the digestive system breaks down the digestible ones into sugar, which enters the blood. As blood sugar levels rise, the pancreas produces insulin, a hormone that prompts cells to absorb blood sugar for energy or storage. Insulin is related to weight gain and that is why you see some people who are overweight later become diabetics.

Some researchers have found that the number of fat cells in your body is set during those pesky adolescence years and remains throughout adulthood, whether you gain weight or lose weight. This is why it is important for people to help their kids, especially during those teenage years. To me, this makes sense. I lost weight in high school and then gained a lot after high school. I have always been able to go back to my high school weight, but no less. The fat cells get bigger with triglycerides and glucose that is taken in. The daily recommended amount of carbohydrates to take in is 300 grams of carbohydrates a day. Some say to lose weight you should take in between 50 and 150 a day. I think when I was losing weight I was probably around 30-50 grams of carbohydrates a day. I did not want to get into ketosis because of the way it made me feel. This is probably why it took me a couple years to lose weight, but I am glad I did it this way. I know a lot of this does not make immediate sense, but there is a YouTube video by Dr. Paul Mason titled "Low Carb from a Doctor's Perspective" that breaks it down in a simple to understand format. This low-carb and high-protein diet is basically the diet I do and it is the opposite of what a lot of people will tell you is the proper human diet. Most people, especially medical professionals, will tell you cut fats and add fibers, where actually you should be adding proteins that do not produce as much insulin and you should be adding fats that produce even less.

*Paleo Diet*

The Paleo Diet typically includes lean meats, fish, fruits, vegetables, nuts and seeds. These are foods that would be obtained from hunting and gathering, if you're into that. Processed foods, sugar, soft drinks, grains, most dairy products, legumes, artificial sweeteners, vegetable oils, margarine, and trans fats are to be avoided. I am not sure what the advantages of this diet is other than taking out preservatives, but someone compared how I eat to the Paleo Diet and I don't see it. I do remember working with one of the military contractors who was doing the Paleo Diet and he was cooking raw vegetables on a wood grill. It did not look very appetizing to me.

## Chapter 3

### See a Doctor! A Good One!

Finding a doctor or a good medical provider should be your first priority before attempting to lose weight. I always liked the provider that I went to and still use him occasionally. He was great at his job and took a lot of time with me, but as his business grew he did not always have the time to sit down and discuss different areas that concerned me or give me advice on many things that I needed to fix. It was a busy rural clinic that saw over 300 patients a day and my provider saw around 60 a day himself. Divide this by a 12 hour shift and that is about five patients an hour. Break that down further and that is 12 minutes per patient, not counting moving between rooms, prepping, and dictation. He once told me that he tries to spend no more than three and a half minutes total with each patient to have an efficient shift. I am not saying this to put him or his business down, just to make you realize that it is hard to find a medical provider, especially a doctor who will sit down and talk to you. My wife worked many years in the medical field and I too worked for several offices setting up training systems and reviewing ways for them to save money. It would surprise you the costs related to medical care and how little the amount of money the providers actually make considering the education required and the amount of liability.

At the end of 2018, as my weight was closing in on 270 pounds, which was about 90 pounds over what I should be, I started to see several health issues arise. My blood pressure was getting extremely high. I was noticing swelling in my lower legs, and I was hearing my pulse in my head at night when I was trying to sleep. Overall, I just felt bad! I've always been able to work around my weight and perform physically, for any task, but now I found that doing common things like working around the yard to even walking up a slight hill was causing me to get out of breath and to sweat profusely.

I went to my regular provider several times for swelling in my lower extremities and one time for chest pains. He put me through about every test and for the first time I was really scared. My main complaint was weight gain and the edema or swelling. I had sonograms of my carotid arteries, EKGs, cardiac stress tests, and even a sleep study.

My blood work came back with low testosterone, low Vitamin D, and high cholesterol. I had a CT-Scan of my chest in which I was told there was a serious issue and he did not call me back after the results came in. That is when I knew I needed to go somewhere else. It ended up being nothing wrong on the CT, but I was stressed mentally for days until I finally got the news. I was never scheduled for a follow-up, even for the issues discovered after the lab results. That is when I definitely knew it was time to find a new medical provider.

My testosterone level was in the 60s, where the normal range is between 250 and 1100 (ng/dL). The only symptoms of low testosterone I was suffering from was extreme tiredness, but I work all the time and did not sleep more than four or five hours a night. I was seeing some issues with mild depression, but attributed this to the lower levels of Vitamin D, which I was running in the low 20s, where the normal range is 30 to 100 (ng/mL). I will discuss Vitamin D in depth throughout the book, but low levels of Vitamin D have been said to cause depression.

I did what is probably the worst thing that someone could do, I tried to self-medicate myself. Luckily for me, my form of self-medicating was with natural over the counter supplements and not illegal street drugs like so many people try. They were not helping, but I thought it was my best option. I started taking 5,000 IU of Vitamin D daily, fish oil supplements (3-6-9), and various non-prescription testosterone boosters that I found online. Not to go into all the details, but most of the online testosterone boosters deal with male sexual performance and that was not one of my symptoms. I spent hundreds of dollars on these things and still felt the same, tired and fat.

One day I was at a Chamber of Commerce event and saw a friend of mine who was working for one of those Male Testosterone Clinics. I am not sure how else to describe it, but that it what they advertise. He was working there and told me that the doctor there was great and could help me with everything. I made an appointment and all seemed great. Blood work showed all the same from before, so he asked me what I wanted. Wow, that was new! A doctor asking me what I wanted. After about 45 minutes I left with a handful of prescriptions, an order for weekly testosterone and vitamin shots, and a promise that I would lose 30 pounds or more in three months. The first couple weeks started off good. I lost 10 pounds and felt better, then it all started falling apart. I started gaining a lot of water weight and was swelling badly in both lower legs. My face felt flush all the time and my blood pressure was well over 150/90 at all times. In fact, on two occasions I was not allowed to participate in training events due to my blood pressure being too high. I started finding excuses to avoid getting my blood pressure taken to avoid not being allowed to work.

Though I was feeling bad, I continued to go in and get the testosterone shots. I never saw the doctor, only a tech who I do not think had any medical training other than in-house training on giving injections. On one occasion I asked to have my blood pressure taken and the tech told me she did not know how and would have to find someone to do it. I asked for blood work and was told that my insurance would not cover it and it would be $300. I later found out insurance did not cover any of the treatments and all were out of pocket in excess of $2,800.00 for just under two months of "treatments and medical monitoring." I finally insisted on testosterone levels being drawn and paid for the test. When I called for the results I was told that I could only get them from the doctor and that the appointment would be $200 in person or $75 by phone, I knew something was wrong. I quit the shots and went back to my poor attempt of treating myself. This was a few months before my wife's surgery which I made the decision to change my life. I was hitting 267 on the scale when I decided to stop weighing myself.

I met my current medical doctor at a charity event. Several people there spoke highly of him and I introduced myself to him and unfortunately he said he was not taking any new patients. I explained what I had been going through and by the end of the night he told me to make an appointment with his office. On my first appointment he told me if my blood pressure did not come down in the next 30 minutes, he was going to call for an ambulance. My blood pressure was 210/104 and I had a bad headache. After about 20 minutes my blood pressure came down enough to continue with the exam. My weight was well over 270 and that was considered morbid obesity by the guidelines for my height of six foot even. He had obtained the lab results from the doctor who gave me the testosterone injections and to all of our surprise, my testosterone was at 1800 and that was over a month after completing the last shot. In fact, all my test results were off in most of the areas of cholesterols, Vitamin D, the B vitamins, etc. If you do an internet search of symptoms of high testosterone in men, I had almost every symptom.

Except for one time in my life, in my early 20s, when I was 280 pounds, I was now the heaviest I had ever been in my life. The doctor put me on blood pressure medicine, which was the first time in my life I'd ever been prescribed a long term medication. Being put on a daily prescription medication put into a bit of mild depression and I realized I was getting old. The medication I took had a diuretic which caused me to lose about eight pounds immediately, but I did not see a reduction in the edema, nor did I see a significant reduction in my blood pressure. Within a couple months, the medication amount was doubled and that was more depressing. The eight pounds I lost in water weight quickly came back because that magical pill that had made me lose water weight did nothing for the overeating, which I was doing. Additionally, I was now taking cholesterol medication, high levels of Vitamin D, and I was given zinc to help flush out the testosterone. We will discuss zinc more in Chapter 8 because it is a very important supplement to take, but like anything, you need good medical direction in doing so.

The cholesterol medication that had been prescribed for me was the worst thing I had ever taken in my life. I got every side-effect listed. I know I sound like a hypochondriac, but I am actually not. I usually try to hide the signs and symptoms of potential ailments hoping they will go away. I do not like going to the doctor, and guess no one really does, but it was my last resort. I was calling in to the doctor's office every couple days and was going in regularly. The doctor agreed to let me discontinue the cholesterol medication, if I could bring the lab numbers down on my own. I started a regular dosage of fish oil, which we will discuss further in Chapter 8. I started walking regularly and it was helping both physically and psychologically to get out. I also started researching various supplements to replace the prescription cholesterol medications and others.

Eventually I was able to come off all the prescribed medications. I make sure my doctor knows all the supplements that I take because there is always a possibility that some supplements will interact with prescription medications and some supplements actually interact with each other. You can also take too much or too little of a supplement and some supplements need supplements to absorb each into your system. I did not know this until asking my doctor about why my Vitamin D lab levels were on the lower scale of normal when I was taking the highest recommended amount of 10,000 IU a day. He told me it needs to be taken with Vitamin K2 for absorption. Sure enough, I looked it up and then was able to find a Vitamin D and K2 supplement and all was good. My Vitamin D level is now in the higher range of normal.

I personally learn best from experience, good and bad. I also learn from hearing other people's experiences. When someone tells me about the best diet to do and what supplements to use, I don't automatically go do it. I look it up, but mostly I listen to people. First of all, people like to be listened to. Have you ever talked to that person who cuts you off or is just waiting for their time to talk? Sometimes I respond with an inquisitive "Really?" Or I just ask a question about what they were talking about. Someone else's experience, good or bad, is research in a simple way. It helps you if you take the time to help yourself.

The internet is a very useful source of diet information, but remember most of those on the internet are not medical doctors or have any medical background at all. There are good sources for various products and tips on specific diets. Over the last two years of exploring different diet plans, I basically stayed with what worked for me, a low-carb and high-protein diet. There are a lot of YouTube channels that specialize in either low-carb or no-carb diets that I get tips from. One in particular is from Dr. Ken Berry who is an actual practicing family medical doctor in Tennessee. Dr. Berry is a good source for the carnivore diet and other low-carb and high-protein type diets. He also has several books about medicine and other subjects related to diets. I have thought about going to see him for medical advice, but due to his location and that with a basic internet search reveals some of the controversies he has been involved in, I decided to watch his videos and learn from there. One good bit of advice that he gives is if your doctor does not take the time to research your questions or is unwilling to consider a low-carb and high-protein diet, then you should consider another doctor. I agree with him on this, but to my disappointment, when my doctor asked me what I was doing to lose weight and I answered that I was doing a modified "keto-style" diet, he said he had never heard of it. I then told him it was like the carnivore diet, with carbs and got another "no" headshake. I then said, "Adkins with carbs." This was followed by an immediate, "That doesn't work." I thought to myself, "Am I the only person doing this?" I was ready to walk out when he started checking my labs and told me that everything looked great, including my cholesterol. There was not a lot of discussion about the diet, but I told him what labs I wanted and he ordered them. For now, he is still my doctor.

You need to educate yourself on what your lab results mean, what labs you should be interested in and what the normal ranges are. Depending on your medical history and family history, there are several areas you should always look at including the good and bad cholesterols, blood sugar levels, proteins, liver enzymes, and other tests that will tell you about cardiac issues and whether or not you could be prone to be diabetic. As you will note, I did not give you the exact tests and that is because I am not a medical doctor. I am passing on my experiences in losing weight, but the information is there for you on the internet. Just be selective and print out questions and take it to your doctor. If they are too busy to listen to your concerns, find another doctor. The health care field is a big business and doctors are humans like anyone else. They have to make money to pay for their office, employees, and insurance to protect them against frivolous law suits. But, they are there to help you and to keep you healthy. If they can't do that, find someone that will.

Hopefully my experiences will help you with your decisions on seeing a good doctor or medical provider.

## Chapter 4

## **Gyms and Trainers**

It is almost like a ritual, when you start a diet you need to join a gym and buy workout clothes. I guess there is nothing wrong with this if you want to spend the money and for most people feel guilty later because you never use that membership. That is what the gyms want you to do. Get that membership that comes directly out of your checking account and when you want to cancel it, well good luck. For this book I joined three different gyms or fitness centers as they like to be called. I joined the most popular one that of course costs the most, the $10 a month chain gym, and a family gym that really wasn't a bad deal at $500 a year for 24 hour access for five family members. It would have been a better deal if we would have used it though.

All the gyms that I joined were good. Of course the one that cost over $100 a month was the nicest with the coolest machines and televisions that you could watch while walking on the treadmill. They had several classes, including a cardio kickboxing class early in the morning. I stuck with it for a few months and did lose some weight, but getting up at 5:00 a.m. to be at a 6 o'clock class got a bit old. Those early mornings meant I had to bring my work clothes with me and would more times than less, forget something and have to rush home before work. So that 30 minute workout was taking up over two hours of my time.

I have always been skeptical over the cleanliness of gyms, especially after the COVID-19 pandemic. I believe that most of them are good about keeping clean, but I had known several people who got MRSA from various contacts at gyms with equipment that was not wiped down by a previous user. If you are not familiar with MRSA, it is Methicillin-resistant Staphylococcus aureus and yes, it is as bad as what it sounds. It is a staph infection that is resistant to a lot of antibiotics and can be spread through direct skin to skin contact or if someone with an active wound passes it on through contact on a gym machine that was not cleaned. I will not get into all the details and everyone should research MRSA on their own, but it is the long term result of us taking antibiotics when not needed. Our bodies have now built up a resistant to these bad things due to overuse of antibiotics. That is the basic description of MRSA, but please research this on your own. Most gyms do a good job of trying to keep clean, but you will always be sharing equipment that someone else has sweated on and hopefully was courteous enough to clean.

There is equipment that is unique to each gym or that may take up too much room or cost too much for you to own. I was getting ready for a pre-employment physical abilities test and one of the machines used in that test was a Stairmaster machine that if I bought it new, it would cost anywhere between $3,000 to $6,000. The membership at this particular gym, which was a local gym, was about $500 a year and that was for four family members and gave all of us 24 hour access. It does not have all the classes that the $100 a month gym has and is a lot smaller, but does the job.

Free weights used to be my favorite until I got into my 40's and found how easy it was to injure myself. Especially if I was trying to show that I could still do what I did in my 20's! I do not aspire to be a major bodybuilder like I had some 25 to 30 years ago, but I know a lot of people are into that and yes, it is hard to have a home gym with all the weights and space to store the big plates. Plus, who would hear you drop the weights after a good clean and jerk or whatever it's called! I enjoy the leg press that you add the free weights to and at one time, several 100 pound plates were fun to throw on each side and push up and down. I would also adjust my feet to do a good calve workout and still do on occasion. Just the 100 pound plate thing is a bit much to put on and look tough. I still do it, but not with the same indifference of 20 to 30 years ago.

CrossFit is actually a brand name for a fitness workout that was developed by Greg Glassman in 2000. It is a trademark and there are over 13,000 franchise gyms in 144 countries. There are also many spin-offs from CrossFit or at least those just copying the multi-million dollar routine without wanting to pay franchise fees. The affiliate fees for CrossFit are $3,000 per year per gym and instructor certification costs $1,000 per instructor, per level. There are four levels of instructors and there are CEU requirements for some levels and recertification fees. The affiliation fees have not changed since 2011 as of the writing of this book, but the information is easy to find with a simple internet search. Those gyms that use the name CrossFit also are required to carry insurance and have other specific rules, like no mobile gyms. The reason I am mentioning all this is because depending on where you live, there are very few regulations on opening a gym or the experience and training that it takes to manage one. Even if it is only a two day or 16 hour training to get the basic certificate, at least there is some training for those who are supposed to be training us. And yes, CrossFit does take legal action for gyms using their name without permission or the curriculum. I have tried a variety of CrossFit gyms and possibly the bootleg ones too. It is a good workout, but a little too much impact on the knees for me. Box jumps are something I never cared for, especially if I was carrying a few extra pounds. The workout was intense and the instructors were very motivating, but the injuries always outweighed the benefits. Plus, I hate puking! I don't know how people could like it, but it seemed to be a norm that someone would work out so hard that they would throw-up. They even had the big industrial garbage cans that the instructor magically pulled out of nowhere and thankfully put it in front of the hurling participant. I don't know about you, but I have played every sport possible, been through some of the most rigorous workouts known to man and have been in burning buildings and worse, yet I cannot remember pushing myself so hard that I puked. It seems that some people use this as a measurement of how extreme the workout is, but for me, that is when I want to curl up in a fetal position and lay on the floor. Maybe it is from being in situations that you cannot vomit in a mask or push yourself so hard that you spend even 15 seconds hurling up your least meal or water, but I have learned to regulate myself to stay on track. Even if it is skipping that 99th flying box jump or whatever it may be! With all this in mind, there will not be a section on binging and purging in this book!

I have tried a multitude of workouts while researching this book. There are thousands of branded and trademarked fitness routines out there, not including the online line workouts. On YouTube alone there were around a quarter million programs, before COVID-19. I tried Zumba, which is also a trademarked fitness regimen started by a Columbian fitness instructor based on dance moves. I thought it looked easy until I tried it and was very sore the day after. It was intimidating to go back to class the second time after having to stop so many times during the first class, but I did. As with most workouts that use repetitive routines, you will get better after time and that may lead to a plateau. A plateau in working out is similar to a weight loss plateau. You get to a point that you are stuck on a certain weight or can't anymore weight or make any progress with your workout. Most repetitive workouts lead to muscle memory. For example, my base or most commonly used workout I do is some type of martial arts and sit-ups. I know, you are reading this and saying asking why I would ever have a problem losing weight if I did martial arts and sit-ups. Mostly, sit-ups which are probably one of the most hated exercise routines in the world. As I mentioned before, I was a chunky kid at times and hated Physical Education or P.E. I hated to run and I sweat profusely at any type of physical activity. In elementary school we were introduced to the Presidential Physical Fitness Awards. I can't remember what grade we started this at, but I remember one thing about that first year and that was the sit-ups! For most of the other events you were either running with the herd or it is a single event that even if you failed, the only one who paid attention was the coach who would say "zero...next" as you jumped up on the pull up bar. But not sit-ups! You are paired up with another classmate and a group of you do it while the whole class watches. When I went to elementary school there was no segregation between male and females, meaning that I could be partnered up with a female to hold my sweaty legs during the sit-up portion of this true Hell Week. We were put in two lines to form groups by some type of mathematical equation that only the P.E. Coach could figure out. As the line trickled down I found myself at the end. I could not figure out how this could happen because my name started with "G" and I should have been in the middle where I would fade into all the other students, but no, I was going last. As the line dwindled down, to my next horror I saw that I was going to be paired with the prettiest girl in class, who was also the smartest and whose parents were also the richest. Can it get any worse? Oh yes, it can. My partner, who looked perfect I am sure, did some inhumanly number that I don't remember, but I do remember the whole class of like 100 plus kids counting. Back then, we would have three classes together with one or two coaches. Well, then it was my turn and I was already sweating. Not just a little bit under the arm pits, but through my pants and even my socks which she had to hold on to. Keep in mind, I had never tried to do a sit-up before this. For some reason, I scammed out of practicing them in class, probably because I was still out on the field walking the mile run. The timing was perfect, I was the last one to go, being an odd number, and I was the only one going. The whole class was watching me and the coach started the stopwatch for one minute. I tried in vain, but could not get any farther than a few inches, if that, off the ground with my shoulders. Instead of just stopping the event, the coach started yelling at me like the drill instructor yelled at Private Pyle in Full Metal Jacket. That was the longest minute of my life and from that point on; I practiced sit-ups until I could do them for what seems forever. Even at my highest weight, I could still do a lot of sit-ups and that would keep people from staring at the fat guy trying to sit himself up. I never one that Presidential Physical Fitness Award patch that was given out to the top 15 percentile in front of the entire school, but did get my name on the wall of my middle school for the most sit-ups in one minute and my name was up there for years after I became an adult. I hoped it would be there when my children went, but with all things, there is always someone better than you. I am sure in today's world this activity is not done in schools anymore. The website is down and from what I read, the event has changed names and I am sure everyone gets a participation award. I guess in a traumatic way, it did change my life and I pushed forward to do well, at least for sit-ups because I built up such a muscle memory for them that it has always been easy.

I found that muscle memory is true, even over years of not doing the particular movement. I started karate as that teen age kid in hopes I would not get picked on anymore. I still got picked on, but just kept out of fights after learning to defend myself...life is so strange! I later took up Taekwondo with my daughters and practiced it for close to a decade. My wife and I were watching Cobra Kai, the television series of the Karate Kid movie series and she said, "That would be a good workout for the book." So we started doing Taekwondo together and I found that even though I did not specifically remember a lot of the forms, the movements were easy and I did not feel sore or if I had worked out at all. My wife was very sore after the workout and felt good each day. The muscle memory made it easier for me and caused less resistance than if I were learning a new movement. For those not familiar with Taekwondo and most martial arts in general, forms are choreographed movements involving punches, blocks, kicks, and other techniques to practice balance while moving and executing them. On the subject of martial arts, whether it is Karate, Taekwondo, or whatever style, most people are scared to go not out of fear of being hurt, but out of fear of being embarrassed. For me, it was like the sit-up competition all over again, but you have to push through it. You have to try and try again if you do not succeed. If you did not read my epigraph at the beginning of this book; The Man in the Arena, please do so. While the sit-up thing changed my life at a young age, this did not really take meaning until I was an adult and learned that you will truly never know victory until you have experienced defeat and you will always wonder "what if" if you do not try. Could have...would have...should have will never apply to me because I will always try and try again if I don't succeed. Enough philosophy, don't give up losing weight just because it is not happening fast enough or the way you wish it would. Keep trying!

As I stated, I have a martial arts background. As a kid, I did it not to get picked on, but mainly because there was a gym there and I could work out. My parents were against me taking karate, but since there was a gym there I told them I was lifting weights and paid for it myself. I later did Taekwondo to spend time with my daughters who were going, but noticed the physical conditioning effects of it. As with many martial arts schools, to keep open they ran an afterschool program and did kickboxing for adults at night along with the Taekwondo. I was around 240 at that time and they had a contest to see who could lose the most weight during their summer promotional for kickboxing. Over that summer, or actually 100 days, I lost over 70 pounds. Now, before you go sign up for your local kickboxing class, there are several factors that went along with this. I was practicing for a martial arts tournament and wanted to drop to the lowest weight class possible because it would give me a height advantage. I had just been selected to be a K-9 deputy and the training was 12 weeks long. The police canines are smart and it is the handler that needs the training and conditioning to be able to keep up with the dog. So every morning started with a 6:00 AM three mile on-leash run with the dog and the last 30 minutes was an off-leash "fun-run" for the dog, which basically meant you had to keep up with the dog as he ran the three mile track on his own. The runs for the handlers included full equipment including ballistic vest, gun belt, gun, and a water supply for the canine and not the handler. The rest of the day included tracking work, first aid training for canines, obstacle courses, classroom work, and everything to become certified. After work I would head directly to the 3:00, 4:00, and 5:30 Taekwondo classes and then do the 6:30 and 7:00 pm kickboxing classes. This was every weekday and Saturdays consisted of a morning kickboxing class and afternoon Taekwondo class for higher level belts. All this and I still had to run with the canine, even on my days off. The weight loss did not seem that difficult at that time, but the workout was mandatory for the canine. I know my final weigh in was 167 and I won the weight loss challenge, but lost the martial arts tournament. Never underestimate someone not as tall as you...they can strike areas you will never imagine.

As I continued to work a lot of hours, I could not keep up with the Taekwondo or the kickboxing classes. Most of the time I worked at night and classes were usually scheduled for the regular nine to fivers. The bad part about working a shift that you get off work after midnight is that you really cannot sleep, especially when you first get home. The weight was creeping back up, mostly because of the on-the-go diet of fast food, pizza, Oreo cookies, and soda. I remember getting home one night at close to 3 AM and watching an infomercial on P90X. What a great idea! A workout that I can do at home by playing them on my DVD player. I don't remember the cost back then, but do know I had to make payments on it. All the workouts could be done at home and with the over-the-door pull-up rack, there was no need for heavy weights. The ninety day program was excellent and it started at the right speed for me. At the end, I was in the best shape of my life and could do dozens of flawless push-ups and well over 20 pull-ups at a time. Pull-ups were never something I could do, so take that Presidential Fitness Award!

P90X requires very little room and limited equipment. You can use various dumbbells or P90X has a substitution of using strength bands, but I find the dumbbells to be the best. They make adjustable weight dumbbells, but I prefer to have separate ones for ease of transition between workouts in the single video. When I start, I do not want to stop. I grabbed a padded barstool at WalMart for around $20 bucks and it is used for some of the exercises, plus I stand at my kitchen counter and type on my computer so they have a dual purpose. When I need a quick break I use the barstool to sit down. Standing when typing burns more calories, plus helps your posture. I do a lot of work on my laptop and used to either sit at a desk, the floor, or even in bed. Over the years I built up quite the midsection. The first area I gain weight is in the buttocks, then the love handles, hips, and stomach. These areas are also the last I lose. When you stand up at your computer you can tighten abs and even your gluteus muscles or butt. I work about 20 minutes, unless I am on a roll with something, and then walk around for five minutes. Even if it is only in my office or kitchen, I move around. Finally, P90X has modified workouts for those with knee issues, which I always used. After I lost enough weight, the knee issues were not as much of an issue, but I remained diligent not to have them reoccur. P90X is part of the Beach Body brand and there is an app that you can get all three P90X series plus dozens of other workouts

*So You Want to Lose Weight?*

and tips for around $100 a year. I simply pull it up on my phone or log in and it is great. With the iPhone you can cast it to a smart television that allows it. Beachbody on Demand is what you search for and remember, I do not make a cut from these products, I simply recommend things that have worked for me.

Since COVID-19 and the subsequent closing of gyms for months, many workouts went online and seemed to do very well. Many people found that they actually only needed a few square feet to work out instead of a massive gym facility that is the size of a Wal-Mart. In addition to the online classes, many people rediscovered walking, biking, and other outdoor activities that got them out of their homes and into the fresh air. As for walking, it is one of the best ways to keep fit and sane. You only burn around 500 calories for every 10,000 steps. 10,000 steps is the equivalent of walking about five miles and would take about two hours if you are walking at a casual pace. The good thing is that a six foot tall male weighing around 180 pounds will burn off 1,800 calories a day normally. I don't really count calories because of the high protein and low carb diet I follow, but the calories I burn are from the extra carbs I take

61

in a day that would normally be stored as fat. Whenever you eat something with carbohydrates in it, they are broken down into glucose, which gives you an immediate source of energy. Too much glucose gets stored in the liver as glycogen. Insulin converts the glycogen into fatty acids to be used at a later time or when needed. The fatty acids are circulated to other parts of the body and stored as fat in adipose tissue which is tissue specific for the storage of fat. We will discuss calories, along with other details on carbs vs. calories in Chapter 7, but remember exercise is good. I have tried the protein only method and did not see the results once I added physical activity.

Talking about good old fashioned activity, let's not forget about yard work, sports, your job, and just generally getting off that "adipose storage area" we sit on and doing something. Changes in your lifestyle can be both good for you and mentally fulfilling. Some of the best weekends I have had were staying at home and doing projects around the house. Push mowing your lawn or someone else's lawn is a tremendous workout and lawn work in general gets you moving around, plus it saves you money on lawn services and makes your house look great. Join a local sports league, even if it is bowling, you are doing more than sitting and watching TV. That is unless you go to the bowling alley and eat hot dogs and those giant pretzels followed by a few pictures of regular beer or worse yet, pitchers of margaritas. Walk when you can and take the stairs both up and down. Most smart phones and smart watches have pedometers on them. Use these apps and challenger yourself daily to take more steps than the week before. Just do something other than sit on that couch eating potato chips and dip!

The last thing I am going to discuss in this chapter is personal trainers. These are the people who make a living helping you work out. I never had a personal trainer until I started doing research for this book. One thing I found out quickly is that they are expensive, especially if they are attached to a business or gym. Depending on the area you live in, personal trainers can cost anywhere between $20-50 for 30 minutes. I never had thought of using a personal trainer until I started doing research for this book. The $100 a month gym I joined gave new members a "free" 30 minute personal trainer session. It was a training session, but was actually a sales pitch for personal training. I was impressed with the first session and the trainer, even though he was just out of high school seemed to have some knowledge of proper workout techniques, nutrition, and he actually identified a shoulder injury I had and modified my workouts. I agreed to continue with two 30 minute workouts a week, but made the mistake of not asking the price until they billed it on my credit card. The cost for eight sessions a month was $360 a month or $45 for thirty minutes. Now I have made fairly good money in my life, but not $90 an hour at 19 years old. The first two sessions went well and I felt good, not $90 an hour good, but felt like I was accomplishing something. Then came the third session which I scheduled at 5:30 AM to work around my crazy schedule. I stayed up late the night before and packed all my clothes for work and got up at 4:30AM to be at the gym ready to go by 5:30 AM. Well, 5:30 AM came and then 6:00 AM and no trainer. Finally, at 6:20 AM he came in as I was leaving for work and said he had car problems. Considering his hair looked like it still had pillow impressions in it, I knew he overslept. I cannot stand being lied and would have been tolerant if he would have told me he overslept instead of continuously insisting he had car problems. I finally said show me the flat tire you replaced and then came the part that he did not even own a car and that it was his girlfriend's car and she drove him to work. I finally called him by name and said, "I know your car and can see it parked out there. I am sure the tire is fine and I can tell if you just put it on or not." I then told him to cancel my personal training. The day was filled with continual text messages and phone calls for me not to cancel the personal training to the point I called the franchise manager. Several sales pitches later, I was told the personal training would be canceled, but for the next three months I was billed $360 and was only refunded once. I had to contact American Express and have them stop the payments.

Most gyms require you to pay electronically from your checking account. It is much harder to cancel payments from your checking account than it is to cancel payments from a credit card. I have personally known many people who have owned gyms or have been in management of gyms. There is nothing better than having a member who pays and doesn't show up. Then just before the renewal time comes up, they suck you back in with free offers. I knew someone who literally had been paying for a gym membership for over four years for a gym that was is their home town from another state.

As with everything in your journey to lose weight, find what works for you. If throwing a few hundred pounds of weights on a bar and lifting it is what works for you, then do it! If running on a treadmill for an hour is what works for you, then do it! And if running in circles and jumping till you puke is for you, well do it, but just not around me!

# Chapter 5

## What is our Body Doing to Us?

The human body is truly an amazing thing. There are checks and balances that adjust our bodies to react to a variety of conditions. Where things go awry is when we try to trick our body or the food and drinks that we take in cause our balanced system to react in wrong ways. To understand how to lose weight, there are some functions that we need to learn about. The information in this chapter is from research I have done while listening to a variety of books, various online videos, and our favorite, the internet. The information is my interpretation of the information and you are encouraged to research the information yourself or consult your medical provider.

*Insulin*

Insulin helps control blood glucose levels by signaling the liver and muscle and fat cells to take in glucose from the blood. Insulin therefore helps cells to take in glucose to be used for energy. If the body has enough stored energy, insulin signals the liver to take up glucose and store it as glycogen in

67

the adipose or fat tissues. Insulin issues lead to diabetes and this can be a deadly condition if not controlled. Pre-diabetes is when your blood sugar is higher than it should be, but not high enough for your doctor to diagnose diabetes. Though most don't realize it, more than one-third of the US population is considered pre-diabetic. Pre-diabetes can make you more likely to get Type II Diabetes and heart disease. A proper diet can avoid becoming pre-diabetic and Type II Diabetes. Type I diabetes is due to a medical condition and usually controlled by an insulin regiment. I am not going into this in depth, but if you are not a Type I diabetic or already diagnosed as pre-diabetic or Type II diabetic, control your weight and intake of foods that take in high carbohydrates and sugars. One symptom of diabetes or pre-diabetes is the emergence of skin tags on the body. When my weight was really high I was getting a lot of them on my neck and under my arm pits. As the weight decreased, they went away. The only way to be sure about any of this is a complete physical examination from your medical provider.

## Leptin

Leptin is one of those mystery hormones that few people hear about when attempting to lose weight. Leptin is produced by your body's fat cells. Fat cells use leptin to tell your brain how much body fat they carry. High levels of leptin tells your brain that you have plenty of fat stored, while low levels tell your brain that fat stores are low and that you need to eat. Leptin is a hormone released from fat cells that are stored in adipose tissue. Adipose tissue is basically fat. It is that tissue under skin, around our organs, between muscles, and other parts of the body. Leptin does not affect food intake from meal to meal but, instead, acts to alter food intake and control energy expenditure over the long term. Leptin's primary target is in the brain, particularly an area called the hypothalamus. Leptin is supposed to tell your brain that when you have enough fat stored, you don't need to eat and can burn calories at a normal rate. Leptin is very effective at keeping us from starving, but something is broken in the mechanism that is supposed to keep us from overeating.

Leptin's main role is long-term regulation of energy, including the number of calories you eat and expend, as well as how much fat you store in your body. The leptin system evolved to keep humans from starving or overeating, both of which would have made you less likely to survive in a world of hunting and gathering. If you really think about it, our bodies balance is so delicate. As with the control of our weight as needed to survive, if a person who depends on their physical abilities to survive, if you are overweight you will not be able to perform as well and if you are underweight or lacking from nutrition, you will not be strong enough. We don't think of this as much today because we don't have to run down our food to eat or fight off predators like our caveman ancestors did. For those who are athletes or ones who depend on physical abilities such as firefighters, law enforcement, military, or anyone who may be in physical fights for their lives, a balanced nutrition is needed.

Our body may also react in ways we don't want it to when we are dieting. We have to remember, our body's systems, such as the leptin system were not developed to help us lose weight because we want to look good for bathing suit season, it developed to make us survive. So when we go on those crash diets, your brain then thinks that you are starving and initiates some very powerful reactions to regain lost body fat so you don't starve. This could be a main reason why so many people have the yo-yo effect when dieting. They lose a significant amount of weight quickly only to gain it back shortly thereafter.

This is why I think dieting slowly is the best for you. I see all the time where people say they just lost 30 pounds in 30 days and yes, it irritates me that I don't do that anymore. But, I have kept my weight off for going on three years now and continue to lose at times. My weight loss was gradual with no more than five pounds a month. I don't think my body was scared I was starving, it just adjusted. I eat far less than what I used to and it was not hard.

Leptin is a hormone released from fat cells in adipose tissue. Leptin signals to the brain, in particular to an area called the hypothalamus. Leptin does not affect food intake from meal to meal but, instead, acts to alter food intake and control energy expenditure over the long term. Leptin has a more profound effect when we lose weight and levels of the hormone fall. This stimulates a huge appetite and increased food intake. The hormone helps us to maintain our normal weight and unfortunately for dieters, makes it hard to lose those extra pounds!

## Ghrelin

Ghrelin is closely associated with leptin and is sometimes referred to as the appetite increaser. Ghrelin is released primarily in the stomach and is thought to signal hunger to the brain. One would expect the body to increase ghrelin if a person was not eating enough and it would decrease if they are overeating. Ghrelin levels have been found to increase in children with anorexia nervosa and decrease in children who are obese.

Researchers found that ghrelin levels are high prior to eating, but go down about three hours after a meal, but some research is now showing that the ghrelin levels decrease after just 20 minutes of eating. There is importance to both theories related to the time ghrelin kicks in and curbs your feelings of hunger. First off, whether it takes 20 minutes or three hours for ghrelin to signal your body that it is not hungry anymore, your meal may be finished if you are eating fast food. There are no specific statistics that I could find on the average time people take to consume a fast food meal, but there is research that says that 20% of all Americans consume their food in their vehicle on their way to or from work. Considering almost one in three Americans eat fast food weekly, I would feel comfortable saying the majority are eating their bag of fast food in less than 20 minutes.

As a doctoral candidate I am used to doing research and did a little unofficial research at my local McDonald's. I sat in the parking lot that gave me the view of the drive through and the store exit to the highway. I noticed that the majority of those who were by themselves immediately started eating as they left the pick-up window. Many were rapidly eating before they drove on the highway and I noticed that this particular McDonald's even had a waste receptacle at the drive through exit for those to put their trash in before leaving the parking lot. As I said, this is a very unofficial research which I did during one breakfast, two lunches, and one diner time. At the most I probably saw 75 cars and most ate something before exiting the parking lot. So, considering it may take 20 minutes for the ghrelin reaction to tell you you're not hungry, it wouldn't matter because you already ate and probably want more.

I have always heard that if you eat small portions and eat slowly it will help you feel full quicker and maybe this is why. Either way, try taking a break from eating for about 20 minutes and see if you are still hungry. I found doing this usually keeps me from going back and eating more. As a side note, I have not eaten McDonald's in well over a year. One of my favorite late night snacks was to get a large fry from McDonald's and eat them on the way home from going out. I did get a small fry off the dollar menu during my second lunchtime observation and they tasted awful. The fries tasted like soap and I could not finish them. It just goes to show you that you can get used to anything if you eat it enough and that you can also live without those fries that you one time thought you lived for.

Chapter 6

## Carbs vs. Protein

There are so many diets out there that have differing opinions. In Chapter 2 I gave a quick overview of some of the more popular ones out there today. Some say lower fat and increase fiber and others say eat only proteins and fats and cut out carbohydrates completely. What I say is do what works for you. I found a long time ago that if I keep my protein grams higher than my carbs I lose weight or at least maintain my weight.

Proteins over carbs are nothing new. I remember my high school biology teacher, Mr. McCord, who is actually my neighbor now, telling us back in the late 70's that steak with the fat on it was good for you. Drink plenty of water and it will all slide right out! That was not popular then when Weight Watchers was cutting the fat and Tab and Fresca kept the calories off with sugar-free sodas. I think he was on to something because some forty years later, that is how I am eating and doing great too! By the way, he still looks the same as he did then and is very active.

Proteins consist of amino acids that are strung together to form complex formations. Proteins are more complex molecules and they take longer to break down in the body to produce energy, therefore they are a paced out and last longer than carbohydrates as a form of energy. One way I have personally noticed this is in the intake of "bad carbs" or basically sugary foods. I don't believe in the "cheat days" where you take one day and eat all the bad foods you want, but I am human. I love cheesecake and mostly if it is covered in cherries with that wonderful cherry syrup. Well, one piece from the Cheesecake Factory is 50 grams of carbs. You may think to yourself that is not bad if you don't take in any other carbs that day, but I have actually felt my pulse rise after eating something like this that is high in carbs and contains no proteins. Processed carbohydrates and other additives such as MSG can cause a spike in blood pressure as the body produces more blood flow to move the items throughout the body to disperse them. Embarrassing as it is, I can say there have been times I have gone to my favorite Chinese buffet and ate so much I felt my heart racing for what seemed to be hours afterwards.

So, how do I deal with the sugar cravings and that sweet tooth? Several years ago I was in Korea teaching a military class and the owner of the company gave me a MET-RX Crisp Apple Pie Meal Replacement Bar. Rich Murphy has always been in good shape and his wife was a competitive body builder. Both firefighters by trade, they both live an active lifestyle and eat healthy. For whatever reason that day, we were unable to break for lunch and he offered me one of the bars which are actually very large and more importantly, tastes great! It is the only high protein bar I have ever eaten that does not taste like a "protein bar." What does a protein bar taste like you say? I can't describe it, but you know it when you eat it! These have been my replacement for something sweet when I have the craving and my quick meal replacement when I am in a hurry or wake up late. I also use them when I have hunger pangs. Hunger pangs or hunger pains are when the stomach has contractions when it is empty. Some people mistaken being hunger for hunger pangs and psychologically feel their stomach contracting, but this is when the body needs to eat. When I feel these hunger pangs is the time I use the MET-RX bars and usually keep one with me at all times. I rarely eat more than half a bar a day now, but if I truly feel hungry or know I need some carbs, I simply take a bite of it. I keep it in a sandwich bag to keep it fresh and usually keep it in my vehicle or backpack with my computer.

They sound like a dieters dream come true, don't they? Well here are the negatives. If you are on a true keto diet, there are carbs, sugar, and corn syrup. So, this is probably not an option for you. They also go against my standard of more protein than carbs. In fact, there are 48 grams of carbs and 31 grams of protein per bar. There is also a nice blend of vitamins, but my intake of daily supplements far outweighs the amount in each bar, so I just count it as bonus vitamins. Remember, this is my go to for those quick boosts or times I cannot eat something that is within my plan. So for me, this is much better than what I used to do which was to buy a 3 Musketeers chocolate bar, which of course they now come in packs of two that are cheaper than buying one. I think my MET-RX bar definitely is better than the 46 grams of carbs and 1 whopping gram of protein in chocolate bar.

Another quick fix snack that is good on the go are single serving peanut butter cups. I don't do the natural ones or the ones that are probably good for me, I buy the Jif-To-Go creamy peanut butter cups. They have 11 grams of carbs and 9 grams of protein, but it is a quick fix and I like it. Like I said, I am sure there are better snacks, but it works for me. These two snacks were life savers this Thanksgiving. All year, my family has going along with the way I eat and trying all the new things we see on YouTube so I could put it in the book. This Thanksgiving was my wife's time to make everything she loves and I think they all had massive amounts of carbs! Apple pie, lemon crème pie, stuffing, mashed potatoes, and on and on. I did try some of each and was worried I would be like that alcoholic who has one drink and is on a multi-day binge, but luckily it did not happen. It was difficult, because we had enough food to feed ten times the number of people who were there to eat, so we had left overs all week. Every time I saw the pies, I took a bite of the Apple Crisp bar. I ate a peanut butter cup to avoid some of the breads and ate turkey as each time I wanted other foods. It worked! My weight fluctuated a little bit, but we walked more and I actually met another goal by a few pounds and have been able to maintain it.

Chapter 7

## Bread or Wraps?

For most Americans bread is the demise of any diet. We love bread. There is nothing better than fresh bread or better yet, fresh baked bread or rolls. I could eat a whole package of croissants and I love potato hamburger buns that are slightly toasted to hold in my ¼ pound burger. What I didn't love was 28 to 46 grams of carbs each of those wonderfully fresh buns packed in. I never ate just one burger; I always had two and at times three burgers. Yes, three half pound burger patties, two or three buns, and of course, fries. The protein in the ground beef does equal about 23 grams of protein, but that is far less than the 50 plus grams of carbs I took in with the meal. The condiments also have carbs, but not that many. Ketchup probably contains the most grams of carbohydrates of common condiments on a hamburger. Each tablespoon has about 5 grams of carbohydrates and if you are like me, between the burger and fries, I probably use 5-10 times that amount.

Breaking the bread addiction is one of the hardest parts of a high protein-low carb diet. It is just natural to wrap something in bread and eat it. Let's not forget the rolls and biscuits! Bread is basically loaded with carbohydrates and even the so called "healthy" bread is sometimes the worst offender. For example: whole wheat bread has about 25 grams of carbohydrates per two slices. The manufacturers tell you the fiber makes it healthy, but you have to burn those carbs off first. Listed on the next few pages are a variety of breads and their total carbs. The sources are varied and these are just estimates, but you get the idea.

Common Types of Bread (2 slice serving) and The Carbs:

|  | (Total Carbs) |
|---|---|
| White Bread | 25 |
| Whole Wheat Bread | 25 |
| Rye Bread | 31 |
| Multigrain Bread | 24 |
| Sourdough Bread | 26 |
| Mixed Grain Bread | 24 |
| Marble Rye and Pumpernickel Bread | 25 |

White with Whole Wheat Swirl Bread  25

Reduced Calorie Bread (2 slices serving)

| | (Total Carbs) |
|---|---|
| Wheat Bread | 20 |
| White Bread | 20 |
| Multigrain Bread | 27 |
| Rye Bread | 21 |

Other Bread Varieties (2 slices serving)

(Total Carbs)

| Cracked Wheat Bread | 25 |
|---|---|
| Italian Bread | 20 |
| Oatmeal Bread | 26 |
| Raisin Bread | 27 |
| Wheat Bran Bread | 34 |

Rolls and Buns (1 roll serving)

(Total Carbs)

| | |
|---|---|
| Dinner Roll | 14 |
| Wheat Dinner Roll | 13 |
| Egg Dinner Roll | 18 |

## Rolls and Buns Continued (1 roll serving)

| | (Total Carbs) |
|---|---|
| French Roll | 19 |
| Hamburger or Hotdog Roll | 21 |
| Mixed Grain Hamburger or Hotdog Roll | 19 |

## Assorted Other Breads

| | (Total Carbs) |
|---|---|
| 1 White Pita Bread | 33 |
| 1 Whole Wheat Pita Bread | 35 |
| 1 Plain Bread Stick | 7 |
| 2 slices Garlic Bread | 26 |
| 2 slices Cheese Bread | 25 |
| 2 slices Onion Bread | 25 |
| 2 slices Egg Bread | 38 |

| | |
|---|---|
| 2 slices Banana Bread | 66 |
| (of course I love banana bread) | |
| 2 slices Baguette | 66 |
| 2 slices Ciabatta | 20 |

Here comes the big mistake if you are watching carbs, wraps. Many dieters think if something is on a wrap, then it is healthy. Maybe if it is full of vitamins and other things that are good for you, but in most cases wraps are high in carbohydrates and in some cases higher than the bread you are trying to avoid. Here is a sample list of various types of wraps and the estimated grams of carbohydrates per wrap.

Popular Types of Wraps

The Carbs:

Flour Wraps

| | |
|---|---|
| 1 small (6" dia) | 15.40 |
| 1 medium (7-8" dia) | 23.62 |
| 1 large (10" dia) | 35.94 |
| 1 extra large (12" dia) | 58.54 |

Whole Wheat Wraps

| | |
|---|---|
| 1 small (6" dia) | 15.07 |
| 1 medium (7" dia) | 22.33 |
| 1 large (8" dia) | 29.03 |
| 1 extra large (10" dia) | 39.07 |

Other Common Suggestions

| | Carbs(g) |
|---|---|
| Whole Wheat Tortilla Wrap | 19.00 |
| Multi Grain Wrap | 17.00 |
| White Wheat Wrap | 19.00 |
| Low Carb Wheat Wrap | 14.00 |

I sometimes just find it better to eat the slice of bread, if I must have bread. As I will discuss later, I am maintaining my weight now, or in what some people call maintenance. With this, I take in at least 40 carbs a day. In doing so, I will make my usual hamburger and take one slice of bread, toast it, and cut it in half for the bottom and one for the top. If you are from the south, you are familiar with Publix supermarkets. If not, it is kind of a nicer than your regular chain of food stores, but not overly expensive. There bakery makes a "Chicago Italian Bread" and packages the entire loaf. It is thin sliced, white bread with a very soft and fresh middle. The crust is good and it is 14 grams of carbohydrates per slice. They are about six by three inches and cut in half, make a good toasted bun of sorts to eat the hamburger. I toast the bread just enough to make it a solid base to hold the burger, but the bread is still fresh on the inside. It is kind of like a paddy-melt, if you ever had one. Either way, it is a great alternative and you do not feel like you are cutting yourself back. If you are on a no-carb diet, this is not an option, but it works for me!

# Chapter 8

## Alcohol and Drinks

In general, drinking alcohol and losing weight don't go well together or at least not for me. In general, an ounce of straight vodka, gin, tequila, scotch, rum, and whiskey have basically no carbs and about 100 calories, if you still count calories. If the alcohol is flavored, there may be an addition of carbs and I look up everything on the MyFitnessPal app if I need a quick reference and to get the official carb count. You can also do an internet search and go to the alcohol producer's website or other general internet search. The majority of carbohydrates come in when you add mixers.

My drink of choice was always a Double Vodka-Cranberry Tall. For those not familiar, that is two shots or two to three ounces of straight vodka and it is put in a taller glass (a traditional "shot" in the United States is 1 ½ ounces. In bars and restaurants, when you order a "tall" it is usually double the mixer or about six to eight ounces of mixer. For me, one drink would give me 28 grams of carbs, which is too much. Also, when I weighed more, I drank more because it took longer for the effects of the alcohol to kick in. I don't know if that is a good thing or not, but I still like the taste of a drink every once in a while, but definitely cannot handle my Double Vodka-Cranberry Tall. That is, not unless I am ready to go to sleep immediately after drinking it.

The mixer, which usually is the carb offender, is generally one and a half times the amount of alcohol. One of mine and my wife's favorite drinks is an apple martini that I created myself. It is a wonderful drink that tastes like a Jolly Rancher and packs almost 12 grams of carbs for every four ounce martini, plus the apple slices that we sometimes add. There are substitutes for the mixers, including sugar free and drinks that have no calories or carbs, like water or other like mixers. The low calorie or low carb substitutes still have calories and carbs. For example, the low calorie cranberry juice I substituted for the real one still has 11 carbs for every serving.

Another reason to strive for sobriety or at least cutting back on your alcohol intake is that alcohol lowers inhibitions and judgment when it comes to not eating that whole bag of chips. It's not just your mental self-control that is affected; you are also physiologically wanting to eat by interactions in your body with alcohol. There is evidence that alcohol can influence hormones that make you feel full. For example, alcohol may inhibit the effects of leptin, a hormone that suppresses appetite that was explained at the beginning of Chapter 4. There are other factors that may be in play when it comes to alcohol and weight loss. Some research suggests that alcohol might stimulate nerve cells in the brain's hypothalamus that increase appetite. According to one study, neurons in the brain that are activated by actual starvation, causing an intense feeling of hunger, can be stimulated by alcohol intake.

Low carbohydrate diets will increase the effects of alcohol. If you were accustomed to having several drinks with little to no intoxicating affects, this will drastically change when you are on a strict no or low-carb diet. Your body stores carbohydrates as glycogen and while you are on a low carbohydrate diet are very low levels of glycogen, especially after you have been on it for a while. Low levels of glycogen mean that there are fewer substances in your body to absorb alcohol. Carbohydrates can reduce blood alcohol levels by absorbing it and therefore with a low carbohydrate diet you get intoxicated faster and with more intensity then you were used to in the past. With these factors in mind never drive, even if you are only having one drink. I have literally felt the effects of alcohol after just one drink because it goes straight into my system with nothing to absorb it. Besides the fact that your Blood Alcohol Level could significantly be higher with one drink than you would have previously experienced leading to a DUI arrest, you could hurt or kill yourself, your family, or someone else. Additionally, if you go out make sure you are with someone you trust that can get you home safely if you get intoxicated. Trust me, the effects of alcohol are strongly intensified while on a low-carb diet.

If having a drink is still your thing, and it is still something I enjoy after a long week, here are a few of the ones that I make on occasion that are somewhat lower in carbohydrates than others. Also, I have listed several different varieties of beers with their alcohol content, calories, and carbs listed. The information is from different websites and if you want to be exact, look up each item yourself or contact the maker. I strive to reflect the best information, but we are all human, right?

*Mixed Drinks*

| | | |
|---|---|---|
| Rum | 1.5 ounces (44 ml) | 0 grams |
| Vodka | 1.5 ounces (44 ml) | 0 grams |
| Gin | 1.5 ounces (44 ml) | 0 grams |
| Tequila | 1.5 ounces (44 ml) | 0 grams |
| Whiskey | 1.5 ounces (44 ml) | 0 grams |

*Spicy Bloody Mary (Two Drinks)*

4 ounces Zing Zang Bloody Mary Mix (6g carbs)

2 ounces of Skyy Vodka (0g of carbs)

½ ounce A1 Sauce (3g carbs per tablespoon) (3g carbs)

¼ ounce Worcestershire Sauce (1g carb per 5 ml) (1g carb)

1 teaspoon or 5 ml of Louisiana Hot Sauce (0g carbs)

½ teaspoon prepared horseradish (1g carb)

1 teaspoon of lemon juice (0g carbs)

1 ounce of pickle juice (0g carbs)

2-3 Olives (1g carbs)

TOTAL: 6g Carbs Each Drink

## Wine

### Carbs in Dry White and Rosé Wine

| Wine | Number of Ounces | Carbs |
|---|---|---|
| Champagne | 5 ounces | 1 |
| Dry rosé wine | 5 ounces | 2.9 |
| Sauvignon Blanc | 5 ounces | 3.01 |
| Pinot Grigio/Gris | 5 ounces | 3.03 |
| Chardonnay | 5 ounces | 3.18 |
| Gewürztraminer | 5 ounces | 3.8 |
| Chenin Blanc | 5 ounces | 4.9 |
| Dry Riesling | 5 ounces | 5.54 |

### Carbs in Dry Red Wine

| Wine | Number of Ounces | Carbs |
|---|---|---|
| Pinot Noir | 5 ounces | 3.4 |
| Shiraz/Syrah | 5 ounces | 3.79 |
| Cabernet Sauvignon | 5 ounces | 3.82 |
| Sangiovese (Chianti) | 5 ounces | 3.85 |
| Grenache | 5 ounces | 4 |

| | | |
|---|---|---|
| Petite Sirah | 5 ounces | 4 |
| Malbec | 5 ounces | 4.1 |
| Zinfandel | 5 ounces | 4.2 |
| Burgundy | 5 ounces | 5.46 |

### Beer

I like the taste of beer. To compare it, I never drank coffee, so if I drink coffee, it tasted awful to me. It is probably because I never grew up drinking coffee, just soda. Soda for breakfast, lunch, diner, and anytime else. Beer was a normal drink around my house growing up. My dad drank beer and as far back as I can remember, I was always begging for a drink. I guess now it would be child abuse, but there may be pictures of me floating around in diapers with a beer in my hand. I am sure they were just staged funny pictures, but I do like the taste of it now. Below are my two beers of choice:

Michelob Ultra 2.6g carbs: I have gotten used to drinking this and it is what I now drink if I want a beer.

Coors Light 5.0g carbs: For many years, this was my beer. It does taste different now that I drink Michelob Ultra.

| *Beer Brand* | % | Cal | Carbs |
|---|---|---|---|
| Amstel Light | 3.5 | 95 | 5 |
| Blue Moon  Blue Moon White | 5.4 | 171 | 12.9 |
| Budweiser (U.S)  Budweiser | 5.0 | 143 | 10.6 |
| Budweiser  Bud Light | 4.2 | 110 | 6.6 |
| Budweiser  Bud Ice | 5.5 | 148 | 8.9 |
| Budweiser  Bud Ice Light | 4.1 | 110 | 6 |
| Busch  Busch | 4.6 | 133 | 10.2 |
| Busch Light Busch Light | 4.1 | 95 | 3.2 |
| Busch Ice  Busch Ice | 5.9 | 173 | 13 |
| Clausthaler Clausthaler | 0.4 | 96 | 5.8 |
| Coors Coors Original | 5.0 | 148 | 11.3 |
| Coors Coors Light | 4.2 | 102 | 5.0 |
| Coors Coors Extra Gold | 5.0 | 147 | 10.7 |

| | | | | |
|---|---|---|---|---|
| Coors | Coors NA | <0.5 | 73 | 14.2 |
| Corona | Corona Light | 4.5 | 109 | 5 |
| Edison Light | | 4.0 | 109 | 6.5 |
| Genesee | Genny Light | 3.6 | 96 | 5.5 |
| Genesee | Kipling Lt Lager | 3.4 | 99 | 8.0 |
| Guinness | Guinness Draught | 4.0 | 125 | 10 |
| Guinness Foreign Extra Stout | | 7.5 | 176 | 14 |
| Hamm's | Hamm's | 4.7 | 144 | 12.1 |
| Hamm's | Hamm's Light | 4.1 | 110 | 7.3 |
| Heineken | Heineken | 5.4 | 166 | 9.8 |
| Heineken | Heineken Light | 3.5 | 99 | 6.8 |
| Henry Weinhard's Amber Ale | | 5.3 | 169 | 14 |
| Henry Weinhard's Dark | | 4.8 | 150 | 13.1 |
| H. Weinhard's Hefeweizen | | 4.9 | 128 | 9.2 |
| H. Weinhard's Private Rsv. | | 4.5 | 128 | 9.2 |
| I.C. Light | I.C. Light | 4.2 | 95 | 2.8 |
| Icehouse | Icehouse 5.0 | 5.0 | 132 | 8.7 |

| | | | | |
|---|---|---|---|---|
| Icehouse | Icehouse 5.5 | 5.5 | 149 | 9.8 |
| J.W. Dundee Honey Brown | | 4.5 | 150 | 13.5 |
| Keystone | Keystone Light | 4.2 | 100 | 5.0 |
| Kilarney's | Red Lager | 5.0 | 197 | 22.8 |
| Killian's | Killian's | 4.9 | 163 | 13.8 |
| Michelob | Michelob | 5.0 | 155 | 13.3 |
| Michelob | Michelob Light | 4.3 | 113 | 6.7 |
| Michelob | Amber Bock | 5.2 | 166 | 15.0 |
| Michelob | Hefeweizen | 5.0 | 152 | 11.8 |
| Michelob | Honey Lager | 4.9 | 175 | 17.4 |
| Michelob | Black & Tan | 5.0 | 168 | 15.8 |
| Michelob | Michelob Ultra | 4.2 | 95 | 2.6 |
| Mickey's | Mickey's | 5.6 | 157 | 11.2 |
| Mickey's | Mickey's Ice | 5.9 | 165 | 11.8 |
| MillerMiller Genuine Draft | | 5 | 143 | 13.1 |
| Miller Genuine Draft Lite | | 4.2 | 110 | 7 |
| MillerMiller High Life | | 5.5 | 156 | 11 |

| | | | |
|---|---|---|---|
| MillerMiller Lite | 4.2 | 96 | 3.2 |
| O'Douls | 0.4 | 70 | 13.3 |
| O'Douls    O'Douls Amber | 0.4 | 90 | 18 |
| Olde English 800 | 5.9 | 160 | 10.5 |
| Olde English 800 Ice | 7.9 | 216 | 14.3 |
| Pete's Brewing Wicked Ale | 5.3 | 174 | 17.7 |
| Pete's Brewing Oktoberfest | 5.8 | 189 | 16.9 |
| Pete's Summer Brew | 4.7 | 163 | 15.6 |
| Pete's Winter Brew | 5.2 | 170 | 15.2 |
| Pete's Brewing Helles Lager | 5.0 | 163 | 14.6 |
| Pete's Brewing Red Rush | 5.3 | 170 | 14.8 |
| Pete's Strawberry Blonde | 5.0 | 160 | 13.6 |
| Pittsburgh Brewing I.C. Light | 4.1 | 95 | 2.8 |
| Pittsburgh Iron City Lager | 4.5 | 140 | 10 |
| Red Dog    Red Dog | 5.0 | 147 | 14.1 |
| Redhook    Redhook ESB | 5.8 | 179 | 14.2 |

| | | | | |
|---|---|---|---|---|
| Redhook | Redhook IPA | 6.5 | 188 | 12.7 |
| Redhook | Blonde Ale | 5.4 | 166 | 13.1 |
| Redhook | Hefe-weizen | 5.2 | 155 | 10.9 |
| Redhook | Nut Brown | 5.6 | 181 | 16 |
| Rhinebecker | | 5 | 106 | 2.5 |
| Sam Adams Light | | 4.05 | 124 | 9.7 |
| Shiner Bock | | 4.4 | 143 | 12.5 |
| Shiner Light | | 3.9 | 120 | 9 |
| Sierra Nevada Pale Ale | | 5.7 | 171 | 14.1 |
| Sierra Nevada Porter | | 5.7 | 194 | 18.4 |
| Sierra Nevada Stout | | 6.4 | 225 | 22.3 |
| Sierra Nevada Wheat | | 4.7 | 153 | 13.1 |
| Sierra Nevada Summerfest | | 4.9 | 158 | 13.7 |
| Sierra Nevada Celebration | | 6.6 | 214 | 19.4 |
| Sierra Nevada | Bigfoot | 9.9 | 330 | 30.3 |
| Yuengling | Premium | 4.4 | 135 | 12 |
| Yuengling | Light | 3.8 | 98 | 6.6 |

| | | | | |
|---|---|---|---|---|
| Yuengling | Ale | 5.0 | 145 | 10 |
| Yuengling | Porter | 4.5 | 150 | 14 |
| Yuengling | Lager | 4.4 | 135 | 12 |
| Yuengling | Black & Tan | 4.5 | 150 | 14 |
| Yuengling | Light Lager | 3.6 | 96 | 8.5 |

## Chapter 9

## **Supplements and Vitamins**

The question that I am asked the most by people that notice my weight loss is, "What are you taking?" Most do not believe that I am not any testosterone shots or taking some type of prescription or over the counter weight loss pill. It is not until someone is around me for a day that they see the regiment of supplements and vitamins I take a day. I either carry the bottles with me in a recyclable grocery bag or prep them the day before in sandwich bags. Either way, I make sure I have them with me at all times to take throughout the day. Taking them all at once does not help and usually leads to nausea. Plus, spreading them out gives you the things you need all day. For the most part, it is difficult to overdose on vitamins and you will usually just secrete them out. Your body can only absorb a certain amount and will pass the rest. It is unfortunate that vitamins and supplements are not like fat that is stored in the body until you need it. Research your vitamins and everything you take. Find out what the upper and lower limits are and find out the negative effects. Sometimes too much can be harmful, just the same as too little. Some vitamins need other things to help them absorb better. As you research, you will find that several supplements have the same co-ingredients. Look at these co-ingredients because they may be there to help you absorb or digest the main ingredient. I know that I used to avoid these supplements s that had other additives because I thought they were fillers, but my doctor was the one who told me what they were and that they were many times needed. Research is the key to vitamins and remember, do what works for you.

I usually do not disagree completely with my medical providers, but when it comes to vitamins and supplements I do. I mainly go to my main medical provider, who is an MD. On occasions, I go to a holistic doctor and to an acupuncturist. One of the doctors told me that vitamins do not work and the only way to increase vitamin levels in the body is through direct intake of foods that contain the vitamins. I have taken Nutrition in college as part of the nursing program I went to and one of the projects was to create a daily diet to get one hundred percent of the daily recommended vitamins and mineral. Basically, it was fairly unrealistic unless you could eat a lot of things like liver and overwhelming amounts of fruits and vegetables. As I continually state throughout this book, I am not an expert and I have not conducted any official research, but personally, my Vitamin B and D levels were very low and now they are all in the upper normal ranges. The same goes with testosterone, it is now in the normal level without any testosterone replacements. It may not be a scientific study, but it works for me.

In writing this book I have bought thousands of dollars in vitamins and supplements. Some I still take, some are on the shelf, and many went into the garbage. Revenue from vitamin and nutritional supplement production reached nearly 31 billion dollars in the United States in 2018 and continues to grow. I am sure with people now worried more about their health than ever it will continue to grow. Many of these supplements have no official testing as to whether they work or not. Many are marketed as the "magic pill" to make you lose weight, but I am sorry to say there is not a magic pill because I have tried almost everything. It is not easy to find what works when there is so little official information. One time I noticed my shoulder stop hurting which I injured several years prior. The constant pain that I had from a partial tear went away completely. I had just added a new supplement and thought that was it, but after a few months the pain came back. No idea what stopped it, but I would stop or reduce one supplement and increase another. After a year, my shoulder pain is gone, so I am not adjusting my intake of supplements as much and still trying to figure out what went right! You will have to find what works for you and most importantly, let your medical provider look at your list of supplements. Many medical providers allow you to enter your vitamins and other medications into their system through apps or online. Hopefully they are looking at what you entered to make sure it is correct, not too much or too little, and that it does not interfere or interact with other medications you may be prescribed or take.

*Multi-Vitamin*

Nature's Way Alive! Max3 Potency Multivitamin, High Potency B-Vitamins, No Iron: Alive! Max3 Potency (with NO added iron) contains a diversity of daily essentials, greens, and antioxidants, vitamins A, C, E, and selenium. This multivitamin is made with essential nutrients, and botanicals including: 23 vitamins and minerals; 12 digestive enzymes; 14 greens; 12 organically grown mushrooms; antioxidants vitamin A, vitamin C, vitamin E, and selenium.  Packed with high potency B-vitamins to convert food into cellular energy, Orchard Fruits & Garden Veggies powder blend (200 mg per serving), and nutrients to support bone health, energy metabolism, eye health, heart health, and immune health.

This is my favorite Multi-Vitamin ever and with the amounts of Vitamin B in them, you definitely notice the difference. In addition to the vitamins, there are plenty of other nutrients that keeps me from taking even more pills a day! The downside is the tablets are fairly big and you have to take three a day. I take them with food since they are so potent to avoid any nausea, but sometimes I do take them on an somewhat empty stomach and do not have issues. I have been taking them for two years now and have seen increases in my Vitamin B profile. I have also not gotten any of the common colds or flus in the past two years, which I also personally attribute to the high levels of Vitamin C, plus my daily intake of zinc. The cost is around $21 a month with Amazon's subscription service. Just make sure you have a month's worth stockpiled in case the shipment is late. There are 90 to a bottle, but remember, you take three a day. I notice when I miss a day by late in the afternoon and then feel more pep after taking them. Below are some of the main supplements, which the amount, and the daily percentage value.

DV in the below list stands for Daily Value of Vitamins provided or the percentage comparison to the recommended daily amount.

| Supplement | Amount | DV |
|---|---|---|
| Vitamin A | 2,700 mcg | 300% |
| Vitamin B6 | 43 mg | 2,529% |
| Vitamin B12 | 80 mcg | 3,333% |
| Riboflavin | 20 mg | 1,538 % |
| Biotin | 33 mcg | 110% |
| Vitamin C | 1,000 mg | 1,111% |
| Vitamin D3 | 50 mcg | 250% |
| Vitamin E | 100 mg | 667% |
| Vitamin K | 120 mcg | 100% |
| Thiamin | 20 mg | 1,667% |

| | | |
|---|---|---|
| Pantothenic Acid | 63 mg | 1,260% |
| Choline | 30 mg | 5% |
| Calcium | 325 mg | 25% |
| Iodine | 150 mcg | 100% |
| Magnesium | 130 mg | 31% |
| Zinc | 11 mg | 100% |
| Selenium | 158 mcg | 287% |
| Copper | 0.9 mg | 100% |
| Manganese | 5.8 mg | 252% |
| Sodium | 10 mg | <1% |
| Potassium | 50 mcg | 1% |

*CoQ10*

CoQ10 100mg Enhanced with Coconut Oil & Bioperine: Coenzyme Q10, more commonly known as CoQ10, is a nutrient that occurs naturally in the body. CoQ10 is found in many of the foods we eat including the organ meats. The organ meats are the heart, liver and kidney. Many people do not like the organ meats or psychologically cannot eat them. Some muscle meats also contain CoQ10 including pork, beef and chicken. Fatty fish are also a good source including trout, herring, mackerel and sardine. For those into the vegan lifestyle or eat vegetables, you can get your CoQ10 be eating spinach, cauliflower and broccoli. Legumes don't count as vegetables, but you can get CoQ10 from soybeans, lentils and peanuts. Soybean has a lot of estrogen in them so I try to avoid them and anything high in estrogen. The fruits that contain the most CoQ10 are oranges and strawberries, but they also contain a lot of sugar. Finally, in the nuts and seeds category, sesame seeds and pistachios are your choice.

Most people have enough CoQ10 from their normal diet. I am sure I do since I eat a lot of chicken, but I do take this supplement daily that has 100 milligrams of CoQ10 and 5 milligrams of black pepper or BioPerine, which helps this and several other supplements in absorbing in the body. Additionally, it also contains coconut oil and is certified vegan friendly for those of you who care about that.

CoQ10 has been used to treat many different conditions. There are articles stating that CoQ10 supplements can lower blood pressure slightly. CoQ10 is also used to treat heart failure and other heart conditions, possibly helping to improve some symptoms and lessen future cardiac risks when combined with regular medications, but as with most supplements the evidence is not officially verified by the FDA or many medical journals. Though still controversial, some preliminary evidence suggests that CoQ10 may help to prevent or treat the adverse effects, such as muscle pains and liver problems, of taking statin-type cholesterol drugs. That is where I first started taking it as an added supplement to a natural cholesterol lowering supplement, Red Yeast Rice. I thought at first it was the cause of me not having any more shoulder pain, but that is more joint related than muscular. As with many supplements, there are articles saying it helps reduce future risks of Alzheimer's disease. I find all this skeptical and sometimes wonder if it is a marketing technique. Finally, CoQ10 has also been studied as a preventive treatment for migraine headaches, though it may take several months to work. It has also been studied for low sperm count, cancer, HIV, muscular dystrophy, Parkinson's disease, gum disease, and many other conditions. However, the research has not found any conclusive benefits. Although CoQ10 is sometimes sold as an energy supplement, there is no evidence that it will boost energy in a typical person. People with chronic diseases such as heart failure, kidney or liver problems, or diabetes should be careful using this supplement. CoQ10 may lower blood sugar levels and blood pressure. Doses of more than 300 milligrams may affect liver enzyme levels. As with all supplements, consult your medical provider before using this supplement, especially if you are taking medications.

This product comes in small soft gels and you only have to take one a day. If you are buying them on Amazon.com, it is actually cheaper at the time I am writing this to buy 120 soft gels than to purchase 30. They cost about $20 for a four month supply.

*Vitamin D3*

Vitamin D3 is becoming one of the most popular vitamins and the benefits are stacking up constantly. There is a lot of research on Vitamin D3 compared to other vitamins and supplements. I started taking D3 many years ago, but was never consistent. The first I heard about it was from a mental health practitioner who was discussing how to handle suicidal people. As a law enforcement officer, which I was for 25 plus years, we dealt with a lot of people suffering from depression. As part of a SWAT team, we were constantly exposed to people who were threatening to harm themselves or others. One of the facts I learned during training on dealing with people suffering from depression was that their Vitamin D levels were many times low. As I researched this, I found that the daily recommended amount was much lower that what was really needed. At the time, the daily recommended amount of Vitamin D3 in the diet was around 10 micrograms or 400 IU. The mental health professional said that a minimum of 5,000 IU should be given daily for a person with no signs of depression and up to 10,000 IU for those suffering from depression. I started by taking Spring Valley Vitamin D3 supplement, which I purchased at Wal-Mart for under $5.00. It contains 5,000 IU of Vitamin D3 and there are 400 small soft gels, but no K-2. I guess this would be sufficient if I had bought the K-2 and took them together, but it was easier for me to buy Vitamin K2 MK-7 Plus Vitamin D3 from Amazon for around

$25.00 for a three month supply. I take two a day and they are small capsules and easy to take.

I would have to say one of the most important supplements to take is a good Vitamin D or D3. This is the one I make sure not to forget to take and don't worry if I go over the maximum amount. I probably get around 12,000 IU a day with food and the extra amount included in my multi-vitamin, but I am good with it. If you remember in Chapter __, I talked about taking supplements and consulting your medical provider. My doctor is a big proponent of Vitamin D3 supplements and I am glad he is. He is the one that told me that I need to take it with Vitamin K-2 for it to adsorb properly. Research also suggests Vitamin D promotes the production of vitamin K-dependent proteins. 17 different types of vitamin K-dependent proteins have been identified so far. Vitamin K-dependent proteins are located within the bone, heart and blood vessels. The overall processes may protect blood vessels and may prevent calcification within the vascular wall.

Vitamin D is a fat-soluble vitamin that can be ingested by foods such as fatty fish, dairy products, and eggs, but is mainly synthesized by the skin through exposure to sunlight. The best way to get it is in supplements and some countries in Europe require it to be added to certain foods to ensure everyone gets the highest amount of Vitamin D3 possible. If you live in the states north of the 35th parallel, which is about two-thirds of the United States, you probably do not get enough sunlight in the winter months to keep up the Vitamin D3 you need. It is imperative that you take these supplements of Vitamin D3 with K-2 to not only fight depression, but to fight other ailments and now possibly even to fight off disease and viruses.

Vitamin D3 levels, 25-hydroxyvitamin D, known as 25(OH)D, is measured by a blood test that your doctor can order. The normal range for adults is between 30-100 nanograms/milliliter or ng/mL. In the past two years my levels went from 21 ng/mL in December of 2018 to 81 ng/ML in November of 2020. I attribute this significant increase to supplements since I try to stay out of the sun due to my light complexion, Florida sun, and history of skin cancer. Though I love salmon, I do not eat enough of it to make that big of a jump.

One of the more prominent discussions on the advantages of Vitamin D3 is its ability to improve the immune system. Studies conducted in the US and in Europe prior to the COVID-19 pandemic showed that those individuals with higher levels of Vitamin D3 had reduced occurrences of Acute Respiratory Infections. During the COVID-19 pandemic, there were multiple articles stating that those with lower Vitamin D3 levels had a higher mortality rate and longer recovery time than those with sufficient levels. There also seems to be a relationship between those with certain groups prone to have low Vitamin D3 levels and the mortality rate of COVID-19. These groups include those with dark pigmented skin, older adults above the age of 70, and persons who are obese. Since Vitamin D3 is fat soluble, it gets trapped in the adipose or fat tissue. The more fat, the less available the D3 is to be used and therefore less help with the immune system. Darker skin individuals do not produce D3 from sunlight as lighter skin people do and need supplements to help. If this is not done, then there will be a D3 deficiency. Finally, older people, especially over 70, are three times less likely to produce D3 through the skin and therefore are at more risk of lower levels. All three of these groups are in the high risk for COVID-19.

As with most vitamins and supplements, there is little scientific data proving definite benefits, but Vitamin D3 comes the closest in my opinion. I even look at it in my own non-scientist way when it comes to D3 and depression. The state of Washington was averaging around 1,100 suicides a year in 2018, which is up significantly from its already above average rate. Though there was no specific reason other than mentioning rising gun ownership and a suggested lack of mental health treatment availability, Washington State is a rather rainy state. I have traveled through Seattle many times and been to Ft. Lewis for training for several months throughout the year and there are very few sunny days. It would be interesting to see if low Vitamin D3 levels had any impact on this sad statistic.

The benefits of Vitamin D3 and K-2 together are building daily by reputable sources. I would say if you are not taking any supplements, at least take Vitamin D3 with K-2. Most of your multi-vitamins have it included, but not in sufficient amounts. It is possible to take too much that could possibly lead to too much calcium in your system, so consult your medical provider before taking any supplement. But, research Vitamin D-3 online and even on YouTube.com. There are some very informative videos about Vitamin D3, but just keep in mind that many times the sources are not medical professionals.

*Fish Oil*

Omega-3 Wild Alaska Fish Oil (1250mg per Capsule) with Triglyceride. Just one softgel contains at least 1037mg of Omega-3 fatty acids from wild-caught Alaska Pollock. Made with AlaskOmega triglyceride fish oil. Provides Essential Fatty Acids EPA and DHA that may help to support your overall health. Salmon oil is best known for being an exceptionally rich source of omega-3 fats. The primary omega-3 fats found in salmon oil are eicosapentaenoic acid (EPA) and docosahexaenoic acid (DHA). Research has linked the intake of EPA and DHA to a variety of health benefits, such as a reduced risk of heart disease, improved brain health, and reduced inflammation. Some studies have shown that taking omega-3 supplements may help manage symptoms associated with certain inflammatory conditions, such as arthritis and heart disease.

Triglycerides are a type of fat found in your blood. Elevated levels of triglycerides have been identified as a risk factor for heart disease and stroke. HDL cholesterol, which is referred to as "good" cholesterol, is known for having a protective effect on your heart health. Research indicates that the omega-3s found in salmon oil may play a role in lowering triglycerides and raising HDL cholesterol, but finding an official study on this is impossible. Triglycerides are measured by a blood test and are shown in milligrams per deciliter or mg/dL. This should be part of your regular physical your medical provider does along with through a cholesterol screening panel. I cannot say specifically it is due to me taking omega-3s, but my triglyceride level has been cut almost in half in the past two years from 191 mg/dL in 2018 to 100 mg/dL in 2020. The optimal triglyceride level is anything below 150 mg/dL and 200 mg/dL and over is considered high. It used to be the blame for high triglycerides solely fell on eating fatty foods like butter, eggs, meats, and other similar foods. Now, according to many online medical sources, sugar and extra calories are also included in the list of triglyceride offenders, According to the mayoclinic.org if you regularly eat more calories than you burn, particularly from high-carbohydrate foods, you may have high triglycerides. Even with this information so readily available online, whenever I eat something with fat on it people always tell me it will raise my triglycerides. A good friend of mine is a vegan. He is also my attorney and I trust anything he says until it comes to my eating. We went to Five Guys Burgers for lunch one day and I got the bunless burger bowl with double the meat and the sides, minus the bready bun. They put this all together in a box for you and they also have lettuce wraps in lieu of the bun. Rob, my vegan friend got a large order of fries and firmly said, "You will die of a heart attack" and continued to say how his cholesterol levels will be perfect compared to mine. I know his eating habits and that he doesn't work out much and quickly bet him mine would be better. Lucky for him, or me, he is not technologically advanced enough yet to pull up his labs on his phone, but when I showed him mine, he stopped talking about it. The key is also input versus output. If you burn it off, you can eat the sugar, but you must burn it off or it will stay with you. Animal fats pass through you when not used, sugars stay and are given affectionate names such as love handles.

Omega-3 fats from salmon oil make a compound called nitric oxide. Nitric oxide stimulates the relaxation of blood vessels, leading to improved blood flow and reduced blood pressure according to some studies. I also take L-Arginine that has a Nitric Oxide Precursor. I have seen a significant lowering in my blood pressure, but I have also lost over 70 pounds which I am sure that helped too.

The following is a summary of information about Omega-3 use while pregnant. The studies, like most on supplements is not verified and you should never take any prescription, over the counter, vitamin, or any supplement if you are pregnant without fully consulting your medical provider. It is said that Omega-3 fats, like those found in salmon oil, are essential for proper fetal development. Children born to mothers who consume fish or take omega-3 supplements during pregnancy typically score higher on cognitive and motor skill development tests than children whose mothers did not consume omega-3 fats. Omega-3 intake by the mother during pregnancy and the child in early childhood are also associated with a lower risk of behavioral problems in the child. Some research indicates omega-3 consumption may also play a role in preventing preterm births. However, the evidence on this effect is mixed and remains inconclusive. Do not take any supplements or vitamins until you consult your medical provider if you are pregnant.

There is information that omega-3 fats are important for brain development in children and preliminary research suggests they may also promote brain health much later in life. Some research suggests it also reduces the risks of Alzheimer's and Parkinson's disease. Omega-fats are also claimed to reduce eye diseases like glaucoma and age-related macular degeneration.

Finally, omega-3 fats are said to help with dieting and digestion. The fats that are not absorbed in the digestive system are passed. This may lead to some stomach cramps if you are not accustomed to the capsules, but the benefits would definitely outweigh any side effects if any of these possible advantages were found credible. The softgels are actually easy to take and for me, I don't get any aftertaste or burping up of fish taste that I had with others. They are a bit more costly than the Wal-Mart brands, but not having the after taste makes the difference. The cost is about $23 for a three month supply, but remember, you only have to take one to get the minimum suggested amount of 1 gram or 1,000 milligrams a day.

## L-Arginine

NOW Foods Supplements, L-Arginine 1,000 mg, Nitric Oxide Precursor, Amino Acid: L-Arginine (from 1,250 mg L-Arginine HCl) 1 g (1,000 mg) per tablet. Arginine is a conditionally essential basic amino acid involved primarily in urea metabolism and excretion, as well as in DNA synthesis and protein production. It is an important precursor of nitric oxide (NO) and thus plays a role in the dilation of blood vessels. What I have read about L-Arginine is that it helps with protein break down and burns fat. I take one tablet at night before I go to bed and maybe it is psychological, but it seems to help with the weight loss while I sleep. Nothing scientific about my comment, but it works for me. I purchase this from Amazon.com and when I see it on sale, I get it. On sale, it will go for around $15 for 120 tablets.

The tablets are big and not the easiest to take if you do not like swallowing larger pills.

*Lysine*

Lysine is an amino acid. Unlike some other amino acids, the human body doesn't produce lysine so it must be taken in through foods. Sources of lysine include meat, fish, dairy, eggs, and some plants such as soy and other legumes.

People use lysine for cold sores and can take 500 milligrams to one gram a day as a preventative or three to four grams a day if they have an outbreak. Cold sores are actually a form of herpes and stay in the body. There are no medical journals or information proving lysine is good for cold sores, but I know my medical provider did tell me to take three grams a day when I got one and it worked for me. It usually cleared up in a day or two.

I do not have a recommended brand of lysine to purchase. I know I had to purchase some on Christmas Day and found it at my local Walgreens for around $18.00 and that was for 300 tablets at 500 milligrams each. Better yet, I got them BOGO or buy one get one free. I am sure there are better quality supplements out there, but I am happy that I found them on Christmas Day.

*Red Yeast Rice*

I do not currently take this because of some of the side effects and long term side effects. I did take it for a while and had no side effects, but the more I read on this supplement the more I decided not to take it. Though with many supplements it is not verified, but Red Yeast Rice is said to lower the bad cholesterol or LDL in the body. It is also said that it gives some of the same negative side effects. Red Yeast Rice is one of the oldest supplements and used extensively in Chinese Medicine and may have a lot of advantages. Please read up on this supplement carefully and consult your medical provider before taking this or any supplement.

*Resveratrol*

RESVERATROL1450: 1450mg per serving. Resveratrol is part of a group of compounds called polyphenols. They're thought to act like antioxidants, protecting the body against damage that can put you at higher risk for things like cancer and heart disease. It's found in the skin of red grapes, but you can also find it in peanuts and berries.

Manufacturers have tried to capitalize on its powers by selling resveratrol supplements. Most resveratrol capsules sold in the U.S. contain extracts from an Asian plant called Polygonum cuspidatum. Other resveratrol supplements are made from red wine or red grape extracts. This supplement I have listed is from Japanese Knotweed extract.

It's gained a lot of attention for its reported anti-aging and disease-fighting powers. I actually heard about it when I started my weight loss journey on an infomercial one Sunday morning on the radio. It almost got me to order the expensive "Red Wine Extract Miracle Pill" that did everything from lower your blood pressure to let you eat anything and not gain weight. My blood pressure was still high then and so was my weight. I even called the "1-800" number with credit card in hand and was thinking $79.00 a month for this miracle pill was a great price and then I started looking up every ingredient and found that I could get a six month supply for under $26.00. I hung up and ordered everything I needed myself. This was the start of my supplement purchasing and I still take one or two resveratrol capsules a day. I am not sure if it does anything, but my blood pressure is definitely down and I feel good. Still, it's important to note that while experts agree that it does have potential, there's still not enough research to confirm its effectiveness. One of the claims is that it reduces the bad cholesterol or LDL. Mine has actually dropped by half in the past two years, which is great, but I also lost 70 pounds and eat a lot different. Actually, I eat a lot of fatty meats which everyone, including my doctor, told me it would raise the LDL. I am not sure if Resveratrol is the key factor, but I am not taking a chance.

Resveratrol does not have any noted side effects, even in large amounts. It could react with blood thinners if you are taking them so as with any supplement, you should check with your medical provider first. Especially is you are on medications like warfarin or Coumadin and NSAID medications like aspirin and ibuprofen. Even though there are no real studies showing the benefits of resveratrol, since there are no real side effects either, I am going to continue to take it.

*Zinc*

Optimum Nutrition ZMA, Zinc for Immune Support, Muscle Recovery and Endurance Supplement for Men and Women, Zinc and Magnesium Supplement: These are my favorite and my priority daily along with my daily vitamin.

This product is a good combination of three important supplements: Zinc, Magnesium, and Vitamin B6. There is 10.5 mg of Vitamin B6, which helps the body use and store energy from proteins in the foods we eat. B6 is found in foods such as fish and beef liver. It is also found in starchy foods, so it is an important supplement if you are on a low carbohydrate diet that excludes the organ meats. Your body does not produce B6, so you need to take it in through food or as a supplement.

B6 is one of the eight vitamins found in the group of B complex vitamins. The role it plays in the body is still being discovered, but some of the benefits include reducing depression, mostly in older adults. Vitamin B6 may help reduce high homocysteine levels that lead to narrowing of arteries. This may minimize heart disease risk. There are also studies showing other health benefits and you should research it thoroughly.

126

There is 450 mg of Magnesium in each three capsule serving of ZMA. This equals to 107% of the daily recommended requirement of Magnesium. Magnesium is a nutrient that the body needs to stay healthy. Magnesium is important for many processes in the body, including regulating muscle and nerve function, blood sugar levels, and blood pressure and making protein, bone, and DNA.

Very large doses of magnesium can cause serious side effects, including: low blood pressure, irregular heartbeat, mental confusion, changes to breathing, coma, and death. Many articles state that you should limit the amount of magnesium to 350 milligrams a day, which is 100 milligrams less than what is in a day's serving of ZMA. With this said, some sites such as WebMD suggest over 400 milligrams a day for males and over 300 milligrams a day for females. I could not find any information stating exactly how many milligrams a person would have to intake for harmful effects, but I think I would stay cautious on the amount you intake due to the reactions magnesium has with the heart. If you are taking magnesium supplements, as I am, you may want to be careful taking it in from other sources such as food, supplements, or medications. Laxatives, in particular, often contain high levels of magnesium, due to its natural laxative effects. Although these medications provide more than the recommended amount of magnesium, the body usually does not absorb it all. For example, one tablespoon of Milk of Magnesia contains 500 mg of elemental magnesium. A daily dose for adults is up to four tablespoons per day, but the body excretes much of the magnesium because of the medication's laxative effects. Some migraine medications also contain magnesium, as do some drugs for indigestion and heartburn. Only take a medication that contains magnesium with medical supervision and make sure you mention to your medical provider the amounts you intake daily. A suggestion is to have your medical provider add a check for magnesium to your blood draw to find the levels.

I marked these in reverse order of the name, ZMA, because zinc is the most important supplement we can take, besides the essential daily recommended vitamins and minerals. According to the National Institute of Health (NIH), the "adequate" amount of zinc intake a day is 11 milligrams for men and eight milligrams for women. The body does not store or produce zinc in the body naturally, so a daily intake is recommended and I try to take it at least three times a day to make sure I am well above adequate.

Zinc is an essential mineral that is naturally present in some foods and available as a supplement. Zinc is also found in many cold lozenges and some over-the-counter drugs sold as cold remedies. When COVID-19 first emerged, many people, including doctors were recommending high amounts of zinc to prevent and battle the deadly virus. In July of 2020, the NIH said, "Due to its (zinc) direct antiviral properties, it can be assumed that zinc administration is beneficial for most of the population, especially those with suboptimal zinc status." I guess that is about as official as we can get.

Zinc is involved in numerous aspects of cellular metabolism. It is required for the catalytic activity of approximately 100 enzymes and it plays a role in immune function, protein synthesis, wound healing, and cell division. Zinc also supports normal growth and development during pregnancy, childhood, and adolescence and is required for proper sense of taste and smell. I think it is interesting that one of the main symptoms of COVID-19 was the loss of taste and smell. With most supplements, there are not a lot of scientific studies, but there are increases in viral infections in populations that are zinc deficient. With loss of smell and taste a symptom of zinc deficiency, in my non-scientific mind, I see it as a pattern.

It is said that 40 milligrams of zinc a day is the recommended limit. ZMA capsules are 30 milligrams a day total or 10 milligrams per capsule. Some of the research I have seen on zinc says that your body can only process 7.5 milligrams of zinc at a time, so this is a good amount to take. I take it three times a day and spread it between breakfast, lunch, and after diner or at bedtime. I have never had a problem taking it on an empty stomach and they are capsules and not bad to take. They are larger capsules, but after taking some of the others, it is a lot easier. Always check with your medical provider, especially if you are taking large amounts. Research I have looked at does not give the amounts, but there are warnings against large amounts of zinc and using the nasal spray zinc.

Suggested Use: As a dietary supplement take 2-3 capsules daily, preferably on an empty stomach 30-60 minutes before bedtime. For best results, men should use 3 capsules daily. The recommended dosage for women is 2 capsules per day. Avoid taking with dairy or other calcium-containing foods or supplements. I take one capsule with my daily vitamin or just before breakfast, lunch, and diner. Due to the amount of Magnesium, I would not take more than the required dosage.

# Chapter 10

## So What Do I Eat?

The most important thing about eating the right way is meal prepping. There are several options for meal prepping and you can do them according to your diet. An internet search will give you a mind boggling variety of meal preps. I did try one and it was a good variety, but I still had to prepare everything. Read up on these and maybe it was just me, but I want simple. I want microwave to mouth. I want something I can throw in the microwave, heat it up, eat it and keep going. Preferably something I can take with me and keep in a cooler bag or with the least effort possible. Another option is your local restaurants and private meal prepping businesses. When I'm saying local restaurant I am not really talking about take out from Chili's or something like that. Most of your restaurant's foods are packed with carbohydrates or other stuff you don't want. Yes, I did start this book out telling you how I used to eat McDonald's double cheeseburgers and pull the bread off eventually. Well, that does not happen anymore. The burgers are 100% beef according to the McDonald's website, but they are thin and do not have the taste that fresher burgers that you can make at home have. I worked at a McDonald's in the 80's as one of my many side fire department jobs. Firefighters always have second and third jobs on the side, though I don't think many worked at McDonald's. I was clean then and still looks fairly clean. I just like a burger that is about one-third of a pound in weight and I leave it a little pink in the inside so when I heat it up it isn't dry. Over three decades ago, I think there were 10 patties to a pound for regular hamburgers. The food is fine, it just doesn't fill me unless I bought about 10 burgers and threw the bun away, which to me is a waste. There are lists of burger places that will specifically make low-carb meals for you and mainly I will stop at Five Guys because I watch them cook the burgers and I like how they package it. It does cost about $10.00 for a two patties and the sides, but it is filling.

If you do an internet search or social media search of your area you can find a fairly good variety of individuals who do meal preps. I know a few personally and it is a good way to get a custom meal. Some will do your entire day of meals or some will do just a specific meal. There are delivery options to your home or business and I really like the idea of helping someone local with a small business. While writing this book I found out a lot about the local "meal prep" business and that some actually buy from others and mark up the meals and deliver them to you. If someone will not let you come see how they prep the meals, think hard about whether or not you want to eat food that many times is not regulated or inspected. The one I liked the most was about $16.00 a meal for lunch. Still cheaper than going out, but I really do not care about the eating out scene. Food has gotten to be an addition to people and what they plan their life around. There is a phrase that someone told me several years ago, "Eat to live – Don't live to eat." I always keep this in back of my mind.

Finally, what I do is I meal prep at home. Yes, this takes some work, but I will grill about eight hamburgers which will get me through about three days and if I have steak or something else I will grill that too. If it is raining out, which I live in Florida and it rains almost daily, my wife will put the burgers in the air fryer for me. Not the same as the grill, but quicker. My favorite thing to have prepped is chicken thighs. I will buy a large package of thighs with the skin on boil them to cook them through. Remember, you cannot eat raw chicken, it will make you sick. I always do an internet search of how many pounds I have and find out how long to boil them. I then use a meat thermometer to make sure it is done. The internet is the best thing in the world for finding recipes and directions on cooking. If I have time, I soak it for a day in buttermilk to make it tender and more juicy. There are about 12 carbs in a cup of buttermilk, but that is a small amount to me. There are a variety of low carb coatings for chicken, but Shake and Bake for Chicken, the regular one, has about 7 grams of carbohydrates which again, is not too bad for me. I used to fry the chicken in lard and then eat it for several days. Frying in lard is messy and takes a lot of prep and clean up. For the time difference I am happy with the air fryer. Many times I will just have a piece of chicken or a hamburger for breakfast and eat the same for lunch. Keep in mind that I can eat the same thing almost every day, which is a good thing in a low carbohydrate type diet. For those who are not content on the same foods, you should really meal prep in advance. When you are on a high protein and low carbohydrate diet you want to have something to eat to make you full at all times. The chicken is great for me, but you just can't soak chicken and cook it in a minute in the microwave. I find if I am in a hurry what is the easiest to eat, something packaged or worse yet, something through a drive-thru? You have to have your meals planned out. My fall back is on rotisserie chicken or a healthy style deli. Whole Foods or similar type stores will have hot meals or entrees that you can buy as a meal or individually by the pound. This usually works great for me.

There are some foods to watch out for that I found out the hard way. When you think about fish or specifically shellfish you don't expect them to have many grams of carbohydrates. While shrimp and most crabs don't have any carbs or very few carbs, one shellfish that surprised me with the high number of carbs were oysters. I love oysters and will frequently get them raw or slightly steamed. They also come fried which are the best, but part of writing this book was trying different foods and trying to prepare foods that others would like while still maintaining a low carb and high protein diet. One day I prepared the low-carb, high-protein, and semi-healthy pool party for a YouTube video I was shooting to go along with this book. I had low carb beers to sample, different no carb liquors, and low carb mixers. I had other drinks for those who did not want alcohol and two foods that I thought were both southern and low carb; crawfish and oysters. The crawfish were perfect. I bought 20 pounds, which only comes out to around three pounds of actual meat after you peel them, but for every six ounces of meat, that equaled out to around 30 grams of protein and no carbs. Next were the oysters, which I bought 10 dozen or 120 of them still live and in the shell. I bought a "shucking knife set" and had them all ready on ice when I started looking up the carb to protein content to put on little signs for my guests to see. To my surprise each oyster had seven to nine grams of carbohydrates and only about one gram of protein. Now there is a lot of zinc in oysters, around 35 grams for every six medium to large oyster, but the carbs were a huge surprise to me. What is worse is I ate 14 of them while shucking them or opening the shells. Considering I ate the largest ones, just the oysters alone that day put me at 126 grams of carbohydrates when I usually only take in 40 to 50 carbs a day. Everything was a success and the food went over well. We used real butter for the crawfish dip and a lot of hot sauce that is very low in carbs. We had a variety of the seltzer alcoholic drinks that did not go over as well as the Michelob Ultra and other regular beer brands, but we tasted all. After this book and as I am starting my next one on bartending, I will be creating a YouTube channel to companion all my books and give updates on the content. The low carb pool party will definitely be worth watching, especially seeing people who have never had a raw oyster before or sucked the brains out of a crawfish. It is not as bad as it sounds!

Be very careful about what you eat and just because it says "Keto Friendly" it does not mean it is. My life may seem unbelievable at times and I have a lot of different things I do. My career in public safety started off at the fire department in the 1980's and went into the early 1990's when I decided to be a Sheriff's Deputy. I was a deputy, drug agent, K-9 handler, and on the Bomb and SWAT teams for the rest of my career until retiring with a combined 30 years in 2014. Besides getting into politics for the past decade plus in which I wrote my first book "So You Want to Run for Office," that is also available on Amazon.com, Kindle, and Audible.com, I started working at a public safety office in south Florida. It is a combination police, fire, and paramedic job where you work a 24 hour shift and split it between the three jobs doing an eight hour shift in each. It is a great job, but eating can be a challenge. No one there eats the way I do and though they will help me, I still need to plan out my shift for food. Around the holidays people bring food, junk food, to the department. If you look at it from the outside, it looks like a fire department with two rescues, a ladder truck, and engine. In the back are the police cars and everyone is triple certified as police officers, firefighters, and paramedics. So every shift there are cookies, cakes, and my favorite pies left by appreciative citizens of the island community we serve. It is a wonderful thing that people do and I and all the other officers appreciate it. Mostly the others because I don't eat any of the snacks. One day there was some type of chocolate cake with a whipped crème top. The cake itself was super moist and everyone was eating it. To my surprise it said on the label "Keto Friendly." I at first thought it was a joke since firefighters will go to major extremes to play jokes on others, but I looked at another label that gave the business name and social media site. I am not mentioning the name because they are a great business and I would hate to hurt a home based business. I looked at the cake again and knowing most whipped cream isn't too bad in carbohydrates and thought if it is a keto business maybe they found something really low. I finally gave in and tried a small bite of the cake and while it was good and moist, it did not have the texture of regular sugar and carb laden cake, so it must be Keto. I then got a full sized plate and cut piece after piece of the cake and ate it. On the third large piece I started feeling something I had not felt in a while, a sugar buzz. My heart was racing and I thought to myself, this isn't right. I stopped eating and found the store's Facebook page and sent a message to them asking how many carbs per serving and about the protein content. The next morning to my surprise for a Sunday morning I got a response back. It wasn't keto and it was a regular cake. Who knows how many carbs I took in that night, but more than I wanted to I'm sure. The business was very apologetic and even knew the order because someone had them special make it for us. I still secretly think it was one of the other firefighters playing a joke on me and disguised themselves as an elderly couple and delivered the cake just to mess up my diet. The cake was awesome though!

The easiest way to eat is look at the carbohydrates and compare it to the protein. Keep your carbs low and protein high. Stay well under the carb amount you set for yourself. Don't stress over the calories, it is all the carbs, but look for hidden surprises. Net carbs are sometimes the numbers subtracted from proteins. Look at the overall grams of carbohydrates and don't look at net carbs, it will throw you off. Most importantly, always meal-prep and plan your day out. Avoid the crap, and yes I said crap, that is bad for you. Sugars are bad for you and they give you that quick fix, but leave you with regrets later.

## Conclusion

Food is an addiction. Just like anything else in life that you can get addicted to, the problem is that food is everywhere. Food is number one on Maslow's hierarchy of needs. Food gives us energy to live, to work, to play, and to think. If we do not have a balanced food intake we will die. Just like alcohol, tobacco, and other illicit substances we can become addicted to certain types of foods like fast foods, sugars, and just the feeling of having something to eat. When we were children we were rewarded with candy, ice cream, or even getting a "Happy Meal" because it made us happy. People eat to celebrate and they eat when they are down. They eat in large social events and they eat when they are alone. As a society we have become so addicted to food that we have coined a phrase called "comfort food." Comfort food is food that provides consolation, happiness, or a feeling of well-being. Comfort foods typically have high sugar and/or carbohydrate content and are associated with childhood or home cooking.

Prior to the COVID-19 pandemic, the fast food industry in the United States alone was estimated at approximately $2.75 billion, with an even stronger rebound at the end of the pandemic. Soft drink sales in the US have closed in at close to $146 billion a year. Finally, chocolate candy sales in the US alone are over $11 billion annually. Like tobacco and alcohol, the marketing for these items is aimed at continual sales. Children are the targets of sugary cereals and snacks with the use of cartoon figures and advertising during children's shows. Even candy bars come in two packs at a price that makes it "financially irresponsible" to buy a single serving when you can get two for almost the same price. Of course, you never save the second one for later, you eat it then to avoid it from melting or going to waste. In the end it is our responsibility for our own health. Life is full of temptations you just have to make the right choices. Just remember, "Eat to live – don't live to eat."

## About the Author

Jeff Gold is an elected official in Florida, continues to educate himself and works in public safety which he has a lifelong passion for. He spent over thirty years in public safety as a firefighter-paramedic and lieutenant, then later as a supervisor in law enforcement. He continues to work in a public safety agency in south Florida and loves every minute of it. Jeff has associate degrees in both Fire Science and Emergency Medical Services, a Bachelor of Arts in Organizational Studies, a master's degree in Criminal Justice, and has extensive doctoral studies in marketing, business, healthcare management, and is currently finishing his doctorate in education. Jeff and his wife Shawn have five adult daughters; two granddaughters, Skylar Jane and Kinsley Grace; a rescue dog, Puzzle; and Joe the Cat that they rescued from a dumpster. Jeff and Shawn are both very active in their community as volunteers and business owners. Shawn, who is a nurse, has a bachelor's degree in Criminal Justice and owns her own business specializing in medical training, coding, and IT.

## Contact Information

Jeff Gold is the CEO of GSA Services, Inc. GSA Services is a full-service training, logistics, and travel agency that specializes in public safety and military training. Jeff is available for consulting and public speaking on a variety of subjects. If you are a candidate, special interest group, or anyone interested in having Jeff present the information in this book in person, he can be reached at jeffgold@gsaservices.org. Presentations are tailored to your group.

Jeff and his group can also recommend political managers, consultants, and marketing agents at all campaign levels throughout Florida. Jeff is also available for speaking engagements about weight loss.

Please visit our website at gsaservices.org or visit us on Facebook at one of the following pages: So You Want to Run for Office?, So You Want to Lose Weight, GSA Services, Inc., or GSA Travel.

# Other Works

Works Jeff is the author of So You Want to Run for Office? What You Should Know if You Want to Run for Office or Manage a Political Campaign. The book jumps into the truly unknown world of running for office. Jeff has run for public office three times and his last landslide victory was by almost 80% which is almost unheard of in politics. He gives information that most will not give out of fear it will someday be used by someone running against them. It is truly the closest you will come to actually running yourself. It is available in print, on Kindle, and Audible.com.

Jeff and his wife Shawn are the authors of The Bartender's Guide to Drinks: Terms, Tips and Carbs which is the culmination of years of research in bars around the world. Many of the drinks have been passed on to us from bartenders as they made a strange looking drink. We were the couple who passed up the dining area to sit at the bar. Many times the bartender would tell us how to make it and even educate us on the story behind the drink. Sometimes they would just tell us what it is called and others times we were ignored. Others were sent to us and some we just made up ourselves by experimenting at our bar. In addition to recipes there is a section devoted entirely to bartender terminology. Whether you are a career bartender, home bartender, or patron like us, you will know that semi-foreign language that comes from behind the bar. Finally, you will find each recipe has a carbohydrate count and there is a section listing estimated carbs for liquors, beer, wine, garnishes and mixers. You can easily find calories, but for the low-carb and high-protein dieter, this is a rarity. Finally, we list a handful bars we have been to in our section Unique Bars: The Good, Bad and Ugly.

In 2021 look for So You Want to Be a Bartender? Another in the "So You Want to Be" series. This book goes into great detail about the world of bartending with discussions on legal requirements and the tips and tricks of the trade that were barely touched in  The Bartender's Guide to Drinks: Terms, Tips and Carbs book. Look for it in spring of 2021. These books are afternoon readers that allow you to finish the book in two to three hours while holding your attention the entire time. Future subject include law enforcement, firefighting, bomb technicians, and possibly fiction novels.

www.ingramcontent.com/pod-product-compliance
Lightning Source LLC
Chambersburg PA
CBHW060501280326
41933CB00014B/2812